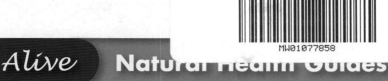

Alive Natural Health Guides

Bee Products
FOR BETTER HEALTH

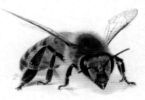

C. Leigh Broadhurst, PhD

Summertown
TENNESSEE

CONTENTS

Introduction 3
Bee Pollen 7
Propolis 18
Royal Jelly 29
Honey 37
Using Bee Products for Healing 53
About the Author 63

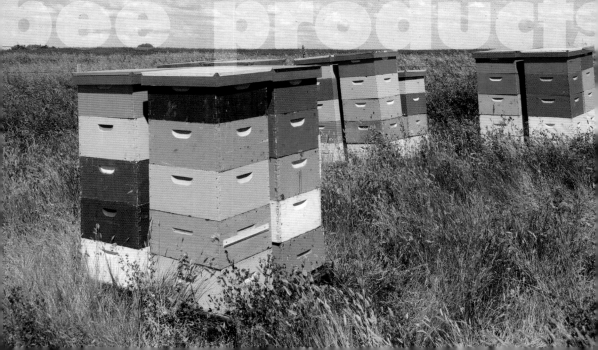

INTRODUCTION

The honeybee (*Apis mellifera*) is the world's most popular insect. Honeybees are fascinating insects because the entire colony essentially functions as one organism. Outdoor workers are responsible for collecting nectar, pollen, and propolis, with different types of workers performing each specialized task. Indoor workers construct and maintain a safe hive and build honey reserves. Nurse bees manufacture royal jelly and tend the larvae and queen, who is solely responsible for female reproduction. Their society is highly complicated and interdependent, just as human society is.

Native to Europe, honeybees have been introduced successfully on every continent except Antarctica. Apiculture (the formal name for beekeeping) has a long history, stretching back to ancient Egypt, Mesopotamia, Greece, Rome, India, and China. According to the US Department of Agriculture, one-third of our food supply depends, directly or indirectly, upon pollination by insects. Bee pollination is worth $16 billion annually to the US agriculture industry alone. Food crops—including almonds, apples, blueberries, cranberries, oranges, peaches, pumpkins, and sunflowers—rely on honeybees for pollination. Alfalfa and clover, also mainly pollinated by bees, are important crops for livestock forage; in addition, these plants are used to revive agricultural fields because their roots harbor symbiotic bacteria that can capture nitrogen (an essential plant nutrient) from the atmosphere and return it to the soil. Bees are big business!

When I was a child my great uncle kept bees in his backyard—once on the outskirts of town, but now in a densely packed suburb of Washington, DC. My grandfather would occasionally take one of his brother's hives and set it up on his farm. It was on my grandfather's farm that I first learned how bees live and how to care for a beehive. I learned how enjoyable chewing chunks of wax comb could be as I savored that fresh, sweet honey straight from the source. Unfortunately, with so much other farmwork to attend to, my grandfather didn't keep his bee colonies going for more than a few years.

When I was a graduate student at the University of Arizona, Tucson, I realized that even on the campus of a major research university, standard medicine had very little to offer people like myself: young, strong, and

ORGANIC BEE PRODUCTS

In order to utilize the USDA Organic seal, bee products must be at least 95 percent certified organic in origin. To determine this, they must be analyzed and found to have acceptably low levels of herbicides, pesticides, and heavy metals. In addition, an area well beyond the bees' source area must be managed using organic methods and certified as such. Products from hives that are used to pollinate conventional crops cannot be labeled USDA Organic.

While the USDA Organic seal is an important indicator of quality, be aware that many apiaries are small businesses that may not have the time or financial resources to become certified organic. This doesn't mean their products are contaminated. One way to ensure purity and high quality in the absence of organic labeling is to look for bee products that come from wild plants.

healthy, but not always able to cope with the stress, late hours, fatigue, poor eating habits, overindulgence in alcohol, and lingering infections that tend to plague students. Then I heard a fascinating interview on a local radio talk show. The guest was Royden Brown, founder of CC Pollen Company, and he was speaking about the benefits of bee pollen. He mentioned beekeepers in Central Europe living to the century mark and beyond without ever having seen a doctor. With sadness I thought of my grandfather, who had died ten years earlier, his body slowly and painfully wasting away with cancer. Meanwhile his brother, the beekeeper, was still going strong, and in fact lived another twenty-five years.

One point that made Royden Brown's interview so compelling was his discussion of how, throughout history, apiculture has provided medicine,

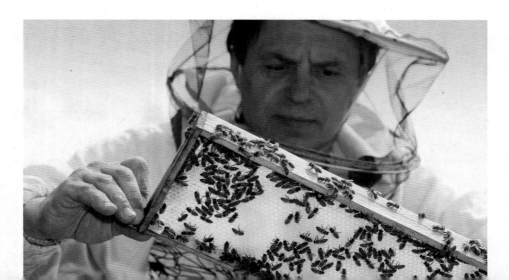

not just food. Beekeepers were among the longest-lived individuals in their villages due to their prodigious use of all the beehive products—honey, propolis, bee pollen, and royal jelly (all four of these will be defined and discussed in the chapters that follow).

I began taking generous doses of bee pollen and propolis every day as part of a quest to maximize my strength and health—a quest that continues to this day. I noticed that these bee products significantly improved my well-being, and perhaps not coincidentally, I polished off my doctoral program ahead of most of my peers. I've since learned that bee pollen is rich in health-promoting phytochemicals. Some of the phytochemicals found in bee pollen can reduce inflammation and promote detoxification. Others are known to lower cholesterol, stabilize and strengthen capillaries, and neutralize free radicals.

I've now spent more than twenty years keeping up with research into beehive products and designing supplements that incorporate them, along with lecturing on the subject. I eat one tablespoon of bee pollen daily, and I'd recommend it to just about anyone. My entire family enjoys pollen, propolis, honey, and royal jelly, and we all support local bee populations by growing extensive vegetable and flower gardens, cultivated without the use of pesticides. I encourage you to do the same, even if you've never gardened. A couple of cucumber plants growing up a trellis will attract bees all summer while also providing you with fresh produce.

Today, rising threats of drug-resistant bacterial and fungal infections and epidemic respiratory diseases have spurred scientific research on traditional medicinal uses of bee propolis and honey—both powerhouses packed with antiviral, antibacterial, and wound-healing qualities. At the same time, bees also face increasing threats. Starting in 2006, large-scale losses of honeybees were reported worldwide. In the United States, beekeepers were losing 30 to 90 percent of their hives per year to a mysterious phenomenon named colony collapse disorder. Despite intense research, no single pathogen, toxin, pollutant, or environmental condition has been shown to cause colony collapse disorder. The best guess is that increasing urbanization has rendered honeybees more susceptible to common bee viruses and parasites, or that an as-yet-unrecognized pathogen has become more virulent.

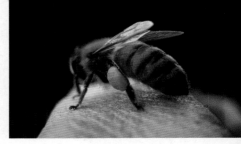

In this book you'll discover a great deal about the healing powers of bee products. For example, you'll learn that propolis prevents disease, royal jelly soothes dermatitis, honey heals wounds, and bee pollen provides copious nutrients. The chapter on honey, which covers the most familiar beehive product, may offer the most surprises. If you think you know honey, think again! Honey has proven its value to skeptics like no other natural product, and if you read the chapter carefully, you'll see why. Honey is still the heart and soul of beekeeping, and by purchasing local honey, you can support local apiaries while also enhancing pollination all around you. In the final chapter of the book, Using Bee Products for Healing, you'll find recipes for home remedies, along with advice on using various bee products for healing.

The theme of this book is that bees are experts in botany, phytochemicals, and medicinal plants. They've spent millennia selecting plants that offer pollen, nectar, and resins that provide superior nutrition while also helping to prevent disease. They've completed thousands of scientific observations to make the most of the plants in their environment, wherever they live on the planet. We just have to learn what bees have to teach us!

A NOTE ABOUT BEESWAX

Although beeswax doesn't have its own chapter in this book, it is a valuable beehive product and worth mentioning. Beeswax is pure, smooth, and clean smelling and has the highest melting temperature of any natural wax. Worker bees secrete the wax from special abdominal glands. Hexagonal wax cells form the structure of honeybee hives. Various cells are used for brood, honey, or pollen storage. The unique honeycomb structure is very strong for its weight and is warm, water repellent, and antimicrobial.

Small amounts of pollen and propolis are partially responsible for the antimicrobial properties of beeswax and provide the unique creamy yellow-brown color. Additionally, the long-chain fatty acids and alcohols that make up the wax are naturally dry and somewhat detergent-like. Thus they don't provide an attractive substrate for most bacteria and fungi to grow.

Today most people encounter beeswax in fine candles. It is also found in waxes used for furniture, leather, skis, and archery equipment, and in shoe polish, soaps, and hair pomades. Beeswax is edible and rarely causes allergic reactions, so it has great value in cosmetics and food protection.

Beeswax is unquestionably the best wax for salves and lip balms, not only because it's nontoxic and edible, but also because it has a remarkable ability to bind with skin's natural waxy sebum, helping to supplement and regenerate the skin. Beeswax also emulsifies well with healing natural oils such as olive, sunflower, and almond. (For an excellent homemade salve, see the Propolis-Beeswax Wound Salve recipe on page 58.)

BEE POLLEN

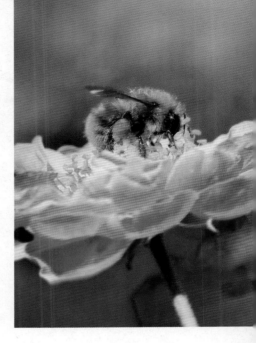

Bee pollen consists of blended pollen grains collected by honeybees from a wide variety of plants. Worker bees travel to hundreds or thousands of flowers daily, collecting pollen in special baskets on their legs. Workers normally collect more pollen than the colony needs, so beekeepers outfit the hives with screens that scrape off some of the pollen as the bees enter. In commercial bee pollen, each of the rounded granules is a bundle collected in a pollen basket on a bee's leg.

Pollen is a major food source for the bees, providing the protein, fat, vitamins, and trace elements (such as calcium, magnesium, iron, and zinc) they require. Plant nectar and honey provide the bees with carbohydrates for energy, but they are not complete food sources. Inside the hive, workers mix pollen with nectar or honey and store it in combs.

Bees that collect pollen are different workers from those that collect nectar. Pollen collectors visit plants that have the most nutritious and easily collected pollen. These plants are not necessarily the same types as those from which nectar is collected.

Widespread use of bee pollen as a food supplement only began around the time of World War II. However, humans have been eating bee pollen as long as they've been eating honey, because raw honey always contains incidental amounts of pollen from the plants from which the nectar is obtained. The characteristic flowery taste of raw, unprocessed honey comes from small amounts of pollen. Processed, filtered honey, on the other hand, contains virtually no pollen.

Bee Pollen: A Highly Nutritious Food

Since pollen consists of the male reproductive parts of seed-bearing plants, it's a very concentrated source of nutrients. The function of the male pollen grains is to fertilize the female ova, resulting in seeds that contain all the genetic material and nutrients needed to grow a new plant.

The nutritional composition of pollen is similar to a combination of dried legumes and nutritional yeast. It can contain 12 to 40 percent protein by dry weight, and its protein contains a complete and balanced spectrum of amino acids, unlike most plant-based foods. This makes it a highly nutritious substance for both mammals and birds.

Pollen contains every vitamin known and is especially rich in nicotinic acid (vitamin B_3), pantothenic acid, and riboflavin (vitamin B_2). Its levels of vitamin B_{12} and vitamin D are fairly low, so pollen is not an adequate source of these vitamins for humans, dogs, or cats.

Over twenty-five trace elements account for 2 to 4 percent of the dry weight of pollen, including every trace element known to be essential for mammals. That said, to use it as a calcium and magnesium supplement you would need to eat about 1 kilogram of pollen per day!

Like most natural whole foods, bee pollen is a healthful choice with respect to dietary fats, with 2 rounded tablespoonfuls of pollen granules containing only 2 to 3 grams of fat. The dominant fatty acids in pollen are alpha-linolenic acid (an omega-3 fatty acid) and linoleic acid (an omega-6 fatty acid), both of which are polyunsaturated; oleic acid, which is monounsaturated; and palmitic acid, which is saturated.

Despite the overall low fat content in the collected pollen, bees apparently seek pollen rich in fats. Fat is crucial to honeybees. They need it to manufacture royal jelly, reproduce, and inhibit the growth of microorganisms in the hive. Dandelion and mustard pollens are some of the richest sources known, with 19 and 11 percent fat, respectively. In contrast, Australian eucalyptus species contain only 0.43 to 4.6 percent fat, with the majority of species containing less than 2 percent. Corn, flax, willow, clover, plants in the cabbage family, and many grasses and fruit trees have pollens that are rich in alpha-linolenic acid.

Bee pollen provides essential nutrients in a concentrated, digestible form. Although vitamin and mineral supplements can provide many benefits, nutrients consumed within foods are superior because they contain a broad range of compounds that work together synergistically. On occasion, people who don't perceive any benefits from standard nutritional supplements find that they improve demonstrably with bee pollen. These people may not be able to absorb and utilize vitamins well unless ingested in the context of a natural food. Bee pollen is also well suited to people who are ill or injured, as they often poorly absorb food and nutrients yet require higher-than-normal levels of nutrients for healing.

The Power of Phytochemicals

Phytochemicals (natural, plant-derived chemicals) are the most important nutritional aspect of pollen—and key to the value of all beehive products. Since pollen is the male reproductive part of a plant, it contains a high concentration of potent phytochemicals to ensure that the resultant seed is viable.

The phytochemical profiles of bee pollen vary, depending on the source plants and their location, the climate, and the season. But no matter where it's collected, pollen is uniformly rich in carotenoids, phenolics and their subcategory flavonoids, and phytosterols.

More than six hundred carotenoids are found in plants. We humans consume about fifty of these in appreciable quantities in our diet, and some of them, most notably beta-carotene, can be converted to vitamin A in the body. Orange, yellow, and red fruits and vegetables, such as apricots, carrots, mangoes, peppers, pumpkin, squash, and tomatoes, are rich in carotenoids. Carotenoids also occur in green produce, but the green pigment of chlorophyll masks them, just as it does in deciduous tree leaves. In autumn, when the leaves of deciduous trees die, the chlorophyll decomposes and the brilliant colors of the carotenoids are revealed. Carotenoids are most valued for their antioxidant properties, but they are also involved in cell-to-cell communication and cell growth.

Phenolic phytochemicals are those based on phenol (benzene alcohol). They are usually soluble in water or alcohol. Every plant has phenolics. Many of them fall into the huge class known as flavonoids, which are widely distributed in food and medicinal plants. All flowering plants contain one or more flavonoids. There are thousands of variations, distinguished by the constituents bonded to the basic flavonoid structure. The most abundant flavonoid in human diets is quercetin.

Phytosterols are part of the steroid group. They have structures similar to animal steroids and some can mimic or regulate human hormones. Steroids are waxy, soapy, or greasy in texture and therefore are more soluble in oil than water. The best-known animal sterol is

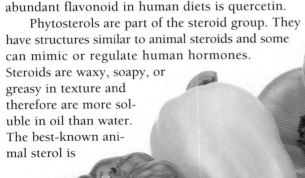

KEY POLLEN PHYTOCHEMICALS

CAROTENOIDS
- beta-carotene
- lutein
- lycopene
- zeaxanthin

PHENOLICS
- anthocyanins
- flavonoids
- phenolic acids
- stilbenes
- cinnamic acids
- isoflavonoids
- polyphenolics
- tannins
- coumarins
- lignans
- proanthocyanidins
- xanthones

FLAVONOIDS
- apigenin
- cyanidin
- kaempferol
- myricetin
- catechin
- genistein
- luteolin
- quercetin
- chrysin
- hesperetin
- malvidin
- rutin

PHYTOSTEROLS
- beta-sitosterol
- brassinosterol
- lanosterol
- stigmasterol

cholesterol—a critical component of our cell membranes, organs, brain, and nervous system, and the precursor for our sex hormones. Analogously, plants are rich in beta-sitosterol, which is a precursor to hormones that control plant growth and reproduction.

Fresh, unheated pollen also contains numerous active enzymes, coenzymes, and hormones, including growth hormones that are at least partially active in humans. It also contains antioxidant enzymes, including catalase, glutathione peroxidase, peroxidase, and superoxide dismutase, which help fight or prevent damage caused by free radicals.

Bee Pollen: The Ultimate Healing Food

The medicinal properties of bee pollen have been appreciated for years. Pollen can help fight anemia, cancer, fatigue, high levels of cholesterol and triglycerides, impotence, infertility, and varicose veins. Since it stimulates the immune system, bee pollen can also aid in recovery from illness and surgery. And because many of the phytochemicals in pollen are antioxidants, it helps combat oxidative stress in the bloodstream and tissues.

All of the health benefits you've ever heard attributed to plant foods can be contained in a single pollen basket.

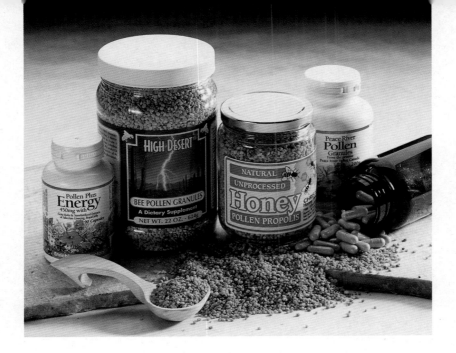

There's hardly a condition that bee pollen cannot help. Bees are phytochemical experts, and they select the best healing compounds that plants have to offer. All of the health benefits you've ever heard attributed to plant foods—from blueberries to broccoli to garlic—can be contained in a single pollen basket. Here are just a few examples:

- The lycopene (a carotenoid) and phytosterols in pollen can reduce prostate inflammation and are associated with lower risk for prostate cancer.
- The strong antioxidant activity of pollen's hundreds of carotenoids and phenolics, unmatched by any other product except for bee propolis, protects against a wide range of health conditions, from heart disease to cancer to cognitive impairments.
- Pollen is rich in flavonoids, including herbacetin, isorhamnetin, kaempferol, luteolin, myricetin, quercetin, rutin, and tricetin. Epidemiological studies indicate that the higher the flavonoid intake, the lower the risk for cardiovascular disease.
- Flavonoids in pollen lower cholesterol, reduce inflammation, and are antibacterial, anticarcinogenic, and antiviral.
- Rutin, a flavonoid that's especially concentrated in pollen, improves the condition and function of capillaries. This helps control diabetic retinopathy, hemorrhoids, hypertension, varicose veins, and venous

insufficiency (a condition in which the veins are unable to pump sufficient blood back to the heart).
- The pollen carotenoids lutein and zeaxanthin help prevent cataracts and macular degeneration.
- Pollen's nutrients and phytosterols improve fertility and reproductive success in animals.

Bees are botanical experts. They've spent millennia locating pollens that are nutritious, abundant, and nontoxic. We just have to learn what they have to teach us!

Bee Pollen, Pollen Allergies, and Hay Fever

Bee pollen can help alleviate allergies, but there's no scientific evidence that it works like allergy shots or that locally derived pollen is required. Wind-borne pollens, which are lightweight and dry to facilitate being dispersed by wind, are responsible for most pollen allergies. The pollens typically harvested by bees, on the other hand, are heavier and sticky so that they'll attach to visiting creatures. They are like microscopic versions of "hitchhiker" burrs that hikers pick up on their socks.

Many well-meaning sources recommend consuming small amounts of bee pollen to provide gradual desensitization to pollen exposure, just like allergy shots. They caution you to consume bee pollen from your local neighborhood, presumably so you're eating the same pollen that's in the air around you. Bee pollen contains only minimal amounts of the wind-borne pollens that are widely allergenic, such as ragweed, birch, olive, and various grasses. Therefore, it simply doesn't make sense to use bee pollen to desensitize yourself to a specific allergen, such as ragweed pollen.

However, there are reasons that bee pollen tends to help improve allergies. Beekeepers primarily select locations for their hives based on access to source plants with nectar that produces tasty, clear honey. Secondarily, they select locations that have access to nutritious pollen source plants that the bees prefer, to keep the colony strong. In general, plants that are known to produce widely allergenic pollen don't fit the criteria used to site beehives, because these pollens aren't adequately nutritious for bees. Flowering plants and bees exist symbiotically, so presumably plants with sticky pollen found it advantageous to produce pollen that keeps bees coming back. In contrast, corn, wheat, alder, hazel, and pine are wind pollinated and produce pollen of inferior nutritional quality. Additionally, quality pollen manufacturers always blend pollen from different locations, seasons, or source apiaries, so there's not a consistent single local source. Such a blend helps minimize sensitization.

Because the phytochemical content in bee pollen supports overall immune health, it can also help fight allergies, even those unrelated to pollen. The large number of antiallergenic, anti-inflammatory, and immune-regulating phytochemicals in pollen are largely responsible for its allergy benefits. The flavonoid quercetin, for example, is antiallergenic, antiasthmat-

Bee pollen reduces allergic symptoms because it is a concentrated source of a variety of plant nutrients and phytochemicals that the human body relies upon and cannot function optimally without.

ic, and antihistaminic, making it valuable in warding off allergies, asthma, bronchitis, chronic obstructive pulmonary disease, colds, flus, and sinusitis. Consuming larger amounts of pollen or allergy preparations containing pollen during hay fever season prevents allergy symptoms more than taking small amounts throughout the year. Using propolis and bee pollen simultaneously helps alleviate allergies more than using either on its own.

As mentioned earlier, bees are phytochemical experts and have been selecting varieties of pollen, nectar, and propolis to keep their colonies healthy for millennia. They purposefully visit a variety of plants, which in turn provide a variety of phytochemicals. Because many of these phytochemicals have similar activities, some redundancy is built in. No matter which pollens are in the blend, it always includes components that will do the job. And when you consume bee pollen, you reap these benefits as well!

Benefits of Bee Pollen for Animals

The majority of bee pollen consumed in North America is eaten by animals. It is added to the diets of piglets, calves, foals, adult horses, rabbits, chicks, laying hens, and pet birds, as it has been shown to enhance growth and overall health, improve fertility, and, in birds, increase egg production. In fact, mice and rats have been shown to thrive on a diet of only fresh bee pollen and water for periods of a month to over a year.

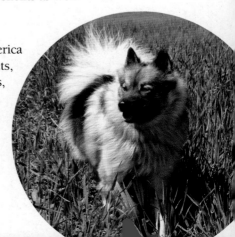

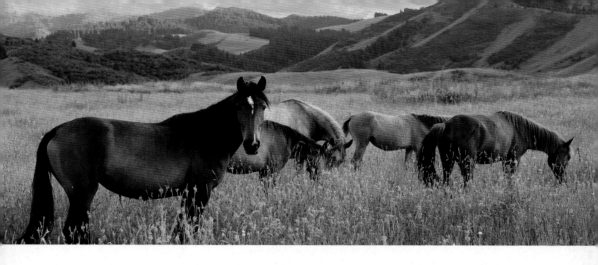

Dogs with poor skin and coat conditions improved when bee pollen was added to their diets.

Racehorses are fed large amounts of bee pollen, particularly on the days just prior to big races. It's a concentrated food source that provides a great deal of nutrients compared to grazing, which not only provides fewer nutrients but also forces the horses to use energy they could otherwise conserve for the race. Horses that were "off their feed"—listless, easily fatigued, and with dull coats—have recovered fully and rapidly when bee pollen was added to their diets.

Horses, cattle, sheep, and goats do eat flowers as they graze, as do wild rabbits and other creatures; therefore, pollen may be an important but overlooked component of their natural, healthful diets. Research has found that domestic rabbits have better reproductive success and ability to handle heat stress when given bee pollen supplements, doing best when they eat 200 milligrams of pollen per kilogram of body weight. Supplementation increased testosterone levels in males and estrogen levels and milk production in females. When rabbit kits were born, offspring from parents fed bee pollen had a better survival rate. Kits grew more rapidly if they were also fed pollen.

Strikingly, rats fed bee pollen had much less body fat than those given chow, and not because they didn't like the meal. When rodents are given chow and bee pollen side by side, they prefer pollen. In similar studies, chicks were observed to preferentially peck out bee pollen granules mixed into commercial bird feed.

Adding pollen to captive birds' diets promotes growth and enhances breeding success. Again, pollen evidently provides dietary components that birds naturally consume in the wild and that are lacking in commercial bird foods or the fruits occasionally fed to captive birds.

Bee pollen is sold in granules, tablets, or food supplements for dogs, cats, rabbits, ferrets, and other small mammals. Cats are obligate carnivores, meaning they can't live or reproduce without consuming animal flesh. Plant foods, including pollen, are not natural components of the feline diet, and cats have a limited ability to metabolize and detoxify phytochemicals. For this reason, cats shouldn't be fed more bee pollen than the manufacturer recommends.

Dogs are more omnivorous than cats, so they can usually handle bee pollen daily. However, too much can cause loose stools in dogs and ferrets, so start with no more than the manufacturer's recommended dose. Rodents can be fed bee pollen in whatever amount and frequency you wish.

Purchasing and Storing Bee Pollen

I recommend high-quality fresh bee pollen, which should consist of soft, pliable granules that haven't been pasteurized or heat-treated. Fresh bee pollen granules are 10 to 20 percent water. Traditionally, pollen is dried in the sun or an oven within days of collection to reduce its water content below 10 percent and inhibit spoilage. However, a better alternative is freezing fresh pollen as it is collected and keeping it frozen until it is vacuum-packed. Freezing retains all the water, resulting in softer, sweeter granules that are superior in taste and nutrition. The granules should smell and taste flowery and sweet-tart, similar to raw honey.

Manufacturers of quality bee pollen always blend pollen from different locations, seasons, or source apiaries. Since some plant pollens aren't as nutritious or tasty as others, it's beneficial to blend sources. Bee pollen from the desert plateaus of the southwestern United States is one of the most nutritious types. Mesquite trees are a major source for this pollen, but many other plants are sampled.

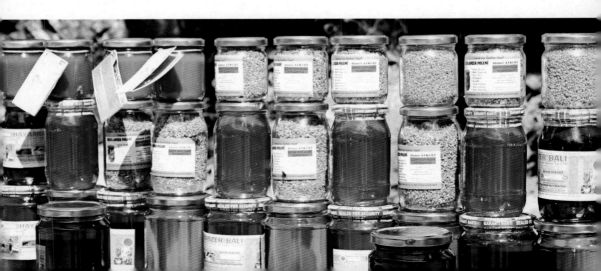

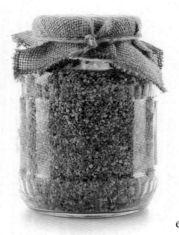

Conscientious manufacturers also utilize bee pollen collected in rural or wilderness areas, away from major sources of agricultural and industrial pollution. The best pollen comes from wild plant sources. Second best but still excellent is pollen from organic farming areas.

Moist, fresh bee pollen will readily grow mold or bacteria if it isn't collected from the screens regularly and dried or frozen within about thirty-six hours. For this reason, pollen collection is more successful in warm, arid areas, such as the southwestern United States and western Spain.

Some processing of pollen is necessary because the pollen grains have two tough outer coats surrounding the nutritive contents. The bees' digestive systems can cope with these coats. Birds and large grazing animals such as horses, goats, and cattle can also handle the pollen coats because they are adapted to processing great quantities of fibrous vegetation and seeds. However, the digestive systems of humans, cats, dogs, pigs, and small mammals cannot break down the coatings. Therefore, better manufacturers gently crack bee pollen before packaging it. This significantly improves the digestibility of the proteins and fats because it allows the contents of the interior to be more easily accessed during digestion, and because some of the proteins and fats are contained in the pollen coats.

Imported pollens are typically subject to oven drying, sterilization, and longer storage, leading to an inferior product. Excessive heating or dehydration of granules gives them a flinty, bitter flavor. Oven-dried and sterilized pollens don't have active enzymes and may also suffer losses of vitamins, polyunsaturated fatty acids, and phytochemicals. In addition, oven drying and sterilization can change the structure of the pollen's proteins. If you detect a sulfurous "rotten egg" odor in bee pollen, it has been overheated to the point where the proteins have degraded.

If you happen to be mildly allergic to bee pollen at first or don't like the quality of a product, don't give up! Instead, please send it back to the manufacturer with a letter indicating that you wish to try a different lot number. You may be sensitive to only one component of the blend, or even to mold spores in the pollen.

Fresh raw pollen should be treated just like fresh produce. Bee pollen sold in plastic bags should be stored in the refrigerator—before and after opening. Pollen sold in jars or cans should always be refrigerated after opening. Any bee pollen product can be stored in the freezer. If you purchase pollen in bulk, put a small refillable container in the refrigerator for daily use and keep the remainder in an airtight container in the freezer. Never add liquids or moist foods to a container of pollen or dip damp fingers or utensils into it. Pollen that is allowed to get wet or contaminated can grow mold or develop off flavors.

Adding Bee Pollen to Your Diet

In terms of phytochemicals, 1 teaspoon of bee pollen is the equivalent of a hearty serving of vegetables. If you're always on the go or know you don't eat all the fruits and vegetables you should, consuming 1 tablespoon of bee pollen daily is a quick and easy way to dramatically improve your diet. Most importantly, you'll be accessing the health-promoting effects of many plants that would not otherwise be part of your diet. It's also a good choice for those who are ill or elderly and perhaps can't cook, chew, or digest large amounts of produce.

When first trying pollen, use fresh, soft granules and take only a few at a time to make sure you aren't allergic to the pollen. If you are allergic to bee stings, be especially cautious about trying any beehive product. Allergies to bee pollen are no more common than allergies to other foods, but they do occur. Sometimes people are highly allergic not just to bee pollen but also to honey, propolis, or royal jelly. Those who are allergic to bee pollen may have multiple pollen and mold allergies. However, most people who are allergic to beehive products are reacting to honeybee proteins. You can be allergic to bee dander just like you can be allergic to cat, dog, or cockroach dander.

If you have no adverse reaction to a small amount of pollen, gradually increase your pollen intake up to 1 tablespoon at a time. A total of 1 to 4 teaspoons per day is a good range for long-term consumption.

Chewing pollen granules or tablets is best way to eat pollen, especially if you're dieting, since you get the full sensation of eating a nutritious food. However, if you can't get used to the taste, mix the pollen with granola, or swallow it whole and follow it with a beverage you like.

Pollen can be added to blender drinks and smoothies, but I don't recommend this unless you really like the taste of pollen and are accustomed to eating it by the spoonful. Similar to citrus zest, a little bit of pollen goes a long way when blended.

PROPOLIS

Propolis consists mainly of resins exuded from the leaf buds and bark of certain trees, collected by worker bees that specialize in resin harvesting. These workers mix the resins with a little wax, honey, and enzymes. The colony uses propolis as putty to seal cracks and openings in the hive and to strengthen and repair honeycombs.

Propolis also helps sterilize the hive, inhibiting the growth of microbes—a significant threat in such humid, close quarters. Some bees practice preventive hygiene by lining brood cells with propolis. It's also used to embalm the carcasses of larger insects and other creatures that have invaded the hive. Intruders such as wasps and mice are quickly stung to death, but the defending bees can't transport heavy corpses out of the hive, so they mummify them to prevent decay.

People have employed propolis as an antiseptic, antimicrobial, and detoxifying agent for both humans and animals for over two thousand years. European, Asian, and Middle Eastern cultures have used propolis to heal festering wounds, such as bedsores, skin ulcers, and jagged battlefield slashes from bayonets. As weapons of war, bayonets are designed to produce wounds that are difficult to suture and don't heal cleanly, thus they readily become infected. These types of wounds particularly benefit from the combination of healing properties in propolis.

Composition of Propolis

Propolis is about 50 percent resins, 30 percent waxes, 10 percent essential oils, 5 percent pollen, and 5 percent plant debris. It's a complex natural substance that contains hundreds of compounds. Chemical analysis of propolis yields a fingerprint of characteristic compounds that often exactly match those in resins collected directly from local trees.

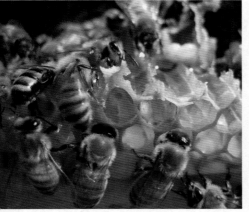

Most research has been conducted on propolis from mixed deciduous and coniferous temperate forests of the midlatitudes of the northern hemisphere. These are the forest types found in northern and central Europe, southern Ontario and Quebec, British Columbia, Canada's Maritime Provinces, and the northern United States. The source trees are mainly poplars, which exude balsam, a sticky resin, from their leaf buds. Resins from beech, chestnut, birch, and aspen trees and various conifers are also harvested. Bees are exceedingly selective; for example, propolis collected in Arizona in the Sonoran Desert contained resin from only a single poplar species: Fremont cottonwood.

Propolis from the United States, Canada, northern and Mediterranean Europe, western Asia, southern Brazil, Uruguay, China, and New Zealand is typically poplar based, with lesser components differing regionally and locally. In northern Russia, propolis mainly incorporates resins from birch and aspen trees.

In tropical South and Central America, Hawaii, Africa, Southeast Asia, and Australia, which have no poplars, honeybees collect propolis from the native vegetation. Studies of Brazilian propolis have identified source trees that include eucalyptus, shrubs in the genus *Baccharis*, evergreen coniferous trees in the genus *Araucaria*, and flowering plants in the genus *Hyptis*. Similarly, Venezuelan bees harvest from evergreen shrubs in the genus *Clusia*. Honeybees were introduced to Hawaii only about one hundred years ago, but they quickly learned to harvest from flowering plumeria shrubs.

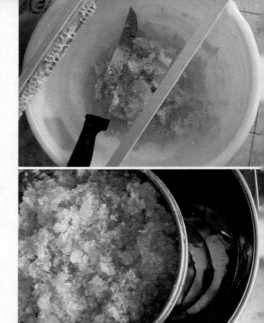

Bees that harvest propolis are phytochemical and medicinal experts doing specialized work for us, gathering and concentrating a unique botanical product that would be too expensive and difficult for humans to collect.

Propolis: A Powerful Botanical Medicine and Detoxifier

Since bees make only minor changes to the resins they collect, propolis is considered an herbal medicine, similar to boswellia, guggul, and myrrh. Despite enormous variation in source plants, most of the medicinal benefits of propolis vary little with origin. Examining propolis from disparate regions—from Chile to Croatia to China—researchers have found a recurrent pattern of antiallergenic, anti-inflammatory, antimicrobial, antioxidant, and detoxifying properties. Most of the compounds responsible for these benefits have been studied in other medicinal plants, but unlike propolis, no plant known contains all of them.

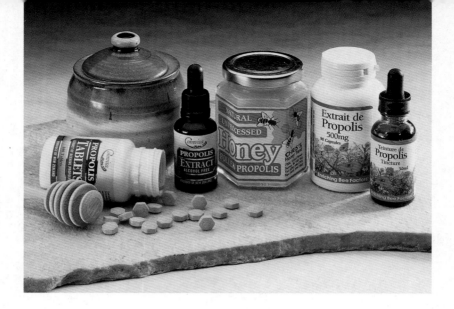

Over two hundred phytochemicals in propolis are known to have biological activity in mammals. Flavonoids are commonly the most abundant compounds in poplar propolis. Among the flavonoids, apigenin, kaempferol, luteolin, and quercetin each possess ten to fifty reported pharmacological and biological properties. Other active flavonoids in propolis include fisetin, galangin, naringenin, pinocembrin, pinostrobin, rhamnetin, tectochrysin, and various hydroxychalcones.

Propolis also contains many types of phenolics other than flavonoids, including benzoic, caffeic, cinnamic, coumaric, and ferulic acids. In addition, it contains essential oil phytochemicals (terpenoids), including limonene, cymene, eucalyptol, and eugenol.

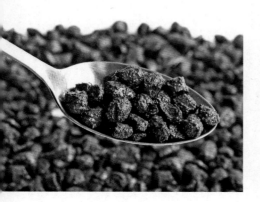

Virtually all day-to-day exposure to toxins is alleviated by antioxidants, discussed in detail in the next section, primarily via enzyme systems concentrated in the liver and skin. We need vitamins and trace elements to manufacture and use these enzymes. The body also detoxifies numerous potentially dangerous or irritating chemicals through reactions with phytochemicals in the diet. This is the primary reason why a high consumption of fruits, vegetables, and bee products (all containing copious quantities of vitamins, minerals, and antioxidants) protects against cancer and many other diseases.

If you are concerned about the effects of environmental chemicals on your health or your family's health, there is no better botanical detoxifier known than bee propolis. For example, three generations of mice fed propolis lived longer than controls fed standard rodent chow. Promotion of detoxification due to better antioxidant protection and liver function was the presumed reason for these benefits.

Propolis: Nature's Premier Antioxidant

By now you're undoubtedly familiar with the phrase "antioxidant protection" in regard to the benefits of eating fruits, vegetables, and other plant foods. Even dog food is fortified with blueberries and cranberries these days. Convenience stores offer pomegranate juice, and kale and collard greens are making a big comeback in recipes. While there's no doubt that higher consumption of produce and herbal supplements promotes health, propolis is a superior source of antioxidants (see the table below). But what is antioxidant protection and why do we need it?

Concentration of antioxidant phenolic compounds in propolis and various produce and beverages

FOOD, BEVERAGE, OR SUPPLEMENT	PHENOLIC CONCENTRATION (in milligrams per gram of food or liquid)
Broccoli	0.35
Spinach	0.4
Cocoa	0.62
Green tea	1
Black tea	1 to 3
Coffee	2 to 2.5
Red wine	2.3 to 3.3
Dates, figs, and raisins	7 to 11
Dark chocolate	12 to 15
Bulgarian propolis	220
US propolis	260
Australian propolis	270
Chinese propolis	300

Oxidative Stress

Both plants and animals create various free radicals, also known as reactive oxygen metabolites, which are unavoidable by-products of metabolism. Free radicals are also created when we're exposed to environmental toxins, drugs, infections, and junk-food diets. Plants need antioxidant protection, just like we do, to keep free radicals from damaging their tissues, and many of the phytochemicals they manufacture serve this function.

Although red wine is purported to be healthful in moderation, it would take six to twelve months of wine drinking to gain the benefits equal to one day's worth of propolis supplements.

Immune system responses unavoidably produce free radicals because, in limited amounts, reactive oxygen metabolites can help kill pathogens and flush toxic substances out of tissues. Free radicals are also produced in immediate responses to trauma, such as cuts, sports injuries, or broken bones—or sliced plant stems. Among other actions, free radicals prompt enzymes involved in damage control, cleanup, and sterilization to begin their work. This causes acute inflammation, warmth, and swelling at the wound site. While this can be painful, it's beneficial because it sets healing processes in motion.

In chronic inflammatory conditions, such as arthritis, tendonitis, asthma, and ulcers, inflammation continues beyond the point where it's beneficial. For some reason, the body just doesn't quit while it's ahead. Chronic inflammatory conditions are characterized by excess

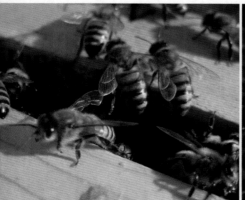
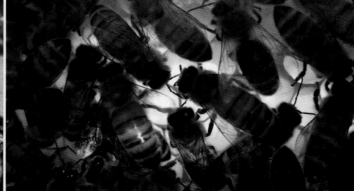

free radicals, which irritate tissues and interfere with healing instead of helping it.

You may be surprised to learn that cardiovascular disease originates in inflammation of the arterial walls. Likewise, oxidative stress is a major factor in diabetes. Chronically high blood sugar levels increase oxidative stress in the body, leading to various symptoms characteristic of diabetes: inflammation of the arteries, hypertension, and visual and nerve degeneration. On a related note, obesity itself can cause chronic inflammation.

Propolis as an Anti-inflammatory

In general, antioxidants help reduce inflammation and oxidative stress, both chronic and acute. Antioxidants act like chemical sacrificial lambs, reacting with and neutralizing free radicals so they don't damage the body's tissues, lessening inflammation, pain, and irritation. Luckily, the antioxidants plants produce to protect their own tissues work equally well for us humans. Therefore, we gain antioxidant protection by eating fruits, vegetables, and honey and taking herbal supplements, including propolis.

Extracts of propolis in ethanol, water, and dimethyl sulfoxide (DMSO) have reliable anti-inflammatory effects in animals and humans. Propolis can help relieve arthritis, asthma, dermatitis, diverticulitis, pustular acne, tendonitis, ulcers, and inflammatory bowel diseases such as Crohn's disease and ulcerative colitis.

One of the major anti-inflammatory phytochemicals in propolis is caffeic acid phenethyl ester (CAPE). High levels of CAPE are unique to non-

Our bodies depend on antioxidant phytochemicals for protection from free radical damage. Without them, we will suffer from chronic disease and lethargy.

tropical propolis. In virtually every cell culture and animal study, CAPE was the strongest antioxidant and anti-inflammatory compound identified in propolis, having a capacity to reduce inflammation equal to that of certain drugs. When CAPE was removed from propolis samples, they no longer had significant anti-inflammatory activity.

However, tropical propolis can confer certain anti-inflammatory benefits. For example, Brazilian propolis and extracts from the shrub *Baccharis dracunculifolia* (often a source for resins in Brazilian propolis) can both prevent gastric ulcers. Caffeic, cinnamic, coumaric, and ferulic acids were the major compounds that protected the stomach lining from developing inflammatory lesions.

Antibacterial Uses of Propolis

Antibiotic drugs were immensely popular in the latter half of the twentieth century. While they can be highly effective and, in some situations, essential, overuse of antibiotics and the resultant mutations of bacteria into resistant strains have created widespread problems. Pharmaceutical companies and doctors have promoted them extensively, and the livestock industry has employed them excessively. Patients have also played a role by demanding these drugs even when they may be ineffective or dangerous.

Fortunately, nutritional medicine offers excellent alternatives that often suffice, including that ever-effective first line of defense: a good offense. Instead of waiting for infections to arise and then using a pharmaceutical approach to kill bacteria, why not reduce the incidence of disease in the first place? When used in this way, propolis can help combat the development and spread of antibiotic-resistant bacteria. The phytochemicals in propolis with known antibiotic activity fall into several categories: organic acids and their derivatives (such as benzoic, caffeic, cinnamic, coumaric, and ferulic acids), terpenoids (such as cineole, cymene, eugenol, and limonene), and flavonoids (such as galangin, pinocembrin, pinostrobin, and quercetin).

Extracts of propolis in ethanol, acetone, DMSO, and water significantly inhibit the growth of many bacteria that cause common human diseases, such as campylobacter, clostridium, *Staphylococcus* (staph), and *Enterococcus faecalis* (formerly considered a type of strep bacteria). Hence, it is effective against many bacterial diseases (including boils, diarrhea, diphtheria, pneumonia, scarlet fever, strep throat) and infections of the ears, the sinuses, the throat, the urinary tract, and wounds. In studies of Turkish propolis, DMSO extracts were more effective than acetone or water extracts. For some species of bacteria, DMSO extracts performed as well or better than conventional antibiotics. Propolis can also heighten the effectiveness of pharmaceutical antibiotics, including chloramphenicol, neomycin, penicillin, streptomycin, and tetracycline.

Studies have shown propolis to be active against bacteria cultured directly from people with upper respiratory infections, including strains resistant to penicillin. In human studies, propolis helped clear acute bronchitis and sinusitis in adults. When children under twelve were treated preventively with propolis, the incidence of respiratory tract infections was reduced by as much as 55 percent. And because the children had fewer days with fever and severe symptoms, they missed fewer days of school.

To breathe more easily and safely on your next airline flight, try a propolis nose or throat spray.

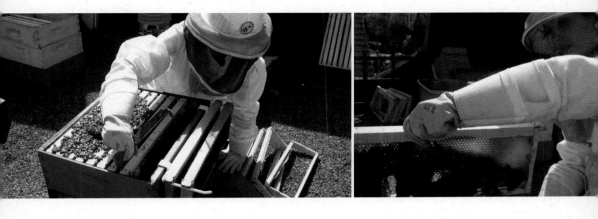

Propolis has more limited activity against *Klebsiella pneumoniae* (which can cause infections of the urinary tract and wounds, in addition to pneumonia) and pseudomonas (which is responsible for many hospital-acquired infections). It is only mildly active or ineffective against *E. coli*, salmonella, and shigella (which causes dysentery).

Antiviral Uses of Propolis

Some of the phytochemicals responsible for propolis's antibiotic activity are also known to be antiviral. Therefore, propolis helps prevent respiratory infections, as most of these infections are caused by adenovirus—the family of viruses often responsible for the common cold. In cell cultures, propolis inhibits replication of other viruses, including those responsible for herpes, influenza, polio, and stomach flu.

Propolis is used to treat genital herpes throughout eastern and Baltic Europe. In a human study, Canadian propolis ointment, acyclovir ointment (a common pharmaceutical treatment), or plain ointment (a placebo) were compared. Lesions treated with propolis healed three to five days faster and were less painful than those treated with acyclovir or placebo.

Propolis for Wound Healing

Everyone suffers minor cuts, burns, and abrasions from time to time. Popular medical opinion and advertising advocate immediate treatment with topical pharmaceutical antibiotics. This approach is flawed, and it's becoming dangerous. This type of frequent casual use promotes the growth of bacterial strains that are resistant to antibiotics.

Research has found that wounds heal faster and more cleanly if treated with propolis. Propolis antiseptic salves prevent the initial growth of harmful bacteria and fungi and have the additional benefit of actually stimulating the healing process, thanks to apigenin, kaempferol, luteolin, quercetin, and other flavonoids that help strengthen tissue and have regenerative effects. In one study, a Brazilian propolis cream was found superior to standard silver sulfadiazine cream in the treatment of minor burns; although both treatments prevented infection, burns treated with the propolis cream healed faster.

The complex blend of compounds in propolis is superior to a conventional ointment containing just one, or perhaps three, antibiotics. It's more difficult for pathogens to develop resistance to complex substances that vary in composition from batch to batch. For example, *Staphylococcus aureus*, which causes wound infections and boils, was cultured with nontoxic levels of propolis extract for forty months, and no resistant strains developed.

Antifungal Properties of Propolis

Trees manufacture resin to protect them themselves from wood-rotting fungi, and those antifungal properties extend to many other types of fungus. Therefore, resin-rich propolis is useful in treating many types of fungal infections, including athlete's foot, ringworm, and most other skin, scalp, and nail fungal infections.

Propolis has also been effective when used topically for vaginal and oral *Candida* infections. Patients with chronic sinusitis caused by *Candida* improved significantly when they sprayed an alcohol-oil emulsion of propolis into their nostrils after daily saline irrigation. However, internal use of propolis isn't reliably effective against chronic systemic yeast infections.

People with AIDS, who have suppressed immune systems, are utilizing propolis for skin and mouth infections, known as thrush, which is caused by *Candida*. This treatment is particularly common in Brazil, where propolis is also taken internally to directly combat the HIV virus.

Note that propolis extracts in propylene glycol, alcohol, or DMSO are useful for treating fungal infections. Extracts in water and especially glycerol are not effective. The compounds in propolis responsible for its antifungal activities include caffeic and coumaric acids and their derivatives; cineole, limonene, and many other terpenoids; and pinocembrin, quercetin, sakuranetin, and other flavonoids.

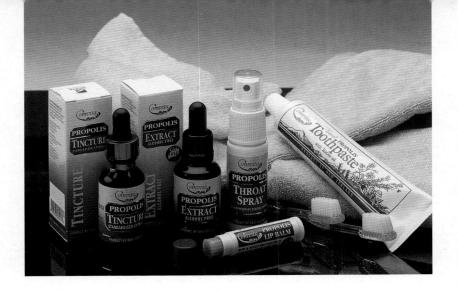

Propolis for Healthy Teeth and Gums

Propolis mouth rinses are astringent and inhibit the growth of common human oral bacteria, which cause gingivitis, halitosis, periodontal disease, and tooth decay. While hydrogen peroxide also effectively kills oral bacteria, it can irritate the teeth or gums and be toxic to the tooth pulp (the living tissue within the tooth). Propolis doesn't have any of these drawbacks.

One of the bacteria controlled by propolis is *Streptococcus mutans*, which creates plaque, an insoluble film of linked sugar molecules that the bacteria secrete in order to adhere to the tooth surface. Propolis also inhibits the growth of other species of *Streptococcus* that have been implicated in cavity formation.

Water-ethanol extracts of European, Indian, Middle Eastern, and Brazilian propolis (0.5 to 5 percent) have been proven effective against bacteria isolated from patients with periodontal disease. These dangerous bacteria proliferate in gum pockets caused by gingivitis and cause infections after oral surgery.

Saliva is naturally protective against oral bacteria; therefore, people with chronic dry mouth have accelerated rates of tooth decay and periodontal disease and will especially benefit from propolis mouth rinses. These rinses also accelerate healing from oral surgery and soothe mouth sores from radiation cancer treatment.

Purchasing and Storing Propolis

Each bee colony harvests propolis from its local area, so the global variation in the plant resins collected is immense. Even within a specific region propolis varies, and some samples are more biologically and pharmacologically active than others. This is intrinsic to the nature of propolis, because it is a botanical product collected in the wild by bees. Choose propolis from a manufacturer that can guarantee the efficacy of the product via laboratory testing, good manufacturing processes, quality assurance standards, and a contact number.

Most of the wholesale propolis in North America is from China, where the costs of the labor-intensive process of producing commercial propolis are reasonable. Chinese propolis from temperate regions has proven as effective as European propolis, but tropical Chinese propolis contains much smaller amounts of active phenolics.

Brazilian propolis generally can't be substituted for other types. It has fewer flavonoids and more terpenoids. Most Brazilian propolis doesn't contain significant amounts of CAPE and therefore may not have the same anti-inflammatory effects. However, Brazilian propolis is effective against bacteria, fungi, and viruses and also promotes detoxification, wound healing, and tissue regeneration.

Suspensions of propolis particles in honey or syrup are readily available and have the advantage of being palatable to children. Propolis suspensions in raw honey are excellent for wounds, burns, and skin infections and, because of their flavor, for children's sore throats.

Use alcohol-based propolis sprays for sore throats and preventing respiratory infections. Use alcohol-based propolis mouth rinses for dental and oral issues. See page 61 for guidelines.

Capsules of powdered propolis are best for detoxification, wound care, and treating chronic inflammatory conditions. See pages 58 and 59 for recipes for salves that include propolis.

Propolis is a fairly stable product. However, to keep all propolis products maximally fresh and effective, store them away from light.

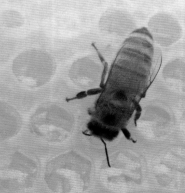

ROYAL JELLY

Royal jelly is the primary food for developing larvae in the beehive. Unlike other hive products, royal jelly is not a plant product collected and modified by bees; it is a substance manufactured by them. Nurse worker bees ingest pollen and nectar and then secrete royal jelly from glands in their heads—a sort of honeybee milk.

All larvae are fed royal jelly for three days. Then the overwhelming majority are cut off because they are destined to become worker bees. Only the queen larvae continue to be fed royal jelly. It is this rich diet consisting solely of royal jelly that transforms the queen into a sexually mature powerhouse, living five to seven years and laying more than her weight in eggs daily. In contrast, worker bees are sterile and live only seven to eight weeks. The queen bee is 40 percent larger and 60 percent heavier than the workers and is fed royal jelly throughout her life.

Fresh royal jelly is roughly 66 percent water, 15 percent carbohydrates, 13 percent protein, 5 percent fat, and 1 percent trace elements. It's a thick, opaque liquid resembling heavy cream.

It contains a complete spectrum of amino acids, either in proteins or free. The carbohydrates are mostly fructose and glucose. The fat fraction contains a mixture of saturated, polyunsaturated, and monounsaturated fatty acids, the latter including linoleic and alpha-linolenic acids. The fat fraction also includes phospholipids, phosphatidylcholine (lecithin) being most abundant. (Phosphatidylcholine, an important nutrient for brain function, particularly in growing children and in the elderly, is also abundant in certain foods, including egg yolks, seeds, and legumes—especially soybeans.)

Royal jelly contains all the B vitamins and is particularly rich in pantothenic acid. It contains lesser amounts of vitamins A, C, D, E, and K. It also contains trace amounts of numerous phytochemicals (mainly flavonoids and phytosterols) derived from the pollen and nectar that the bees use in its manufacture.

While royal jelly is a balanced, nutritious food, it typically isn't consumed in quantities greater than a few grams per day. Sometimes royal jelly is recommended as a complete amino acid supplement for vegetarians or as a source of essential fatty acids. However, because royal jelly is ingested in such small amounts, the protein, carbohydrate, and polyunsaturated fat

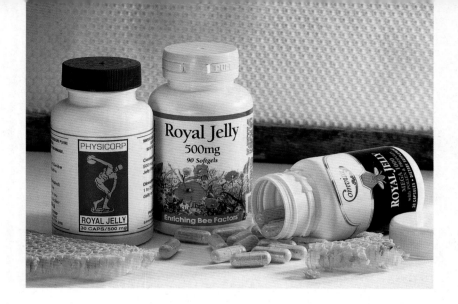

it provides are inconsequential. Rather, it has minor but highly active components that account for its health benefits.

Taking a cue from the beehive practice of feeding royal jelly only to the queen, traditional Chinese medicine recommends royal jelly as a food of the emperors. Considered mysterious and exotic, royal jelly was believed to prolong life, prevent disease, and return the vitality of youth to the aged. It remains prized by modern Asian cultures.

Although we don't know for sure whether royal jelly prolongs human life, a steady diet of it increases the survival rate of mice to old age by 25 percent. In addition, mice trained to swim laps had more endurance and a faster recovery after swimming when fed royal jelly. A reduction in oxidative stress is probably the major reason why mice fed royal jelly had more vitality.

Royal jelly contains all the B vitamins and is particularly rich in pantothenic acid.

Royal jelly is not produced in abundance in the beehive like honey is, and it is expensive and labor-intensive to harvest. Because natural products are used extensively for primary health care in China, and because labor is inexpensive there, royal jelly production is big business in China. Australia, Japan, Korea, and Taiwan also have large royal jelly industries. Unlike honey and bee pollen, almost all royal jelly sold in North America is imported.

Composition of Royal Jelly

Although royal jelly contains many minor components that haven't been fully identified, it's no longer a "mystery" food. We now know that the trace constituents in royal jelly work synergistically with its nutritious base to turn an ordinary larva into a queen. Most notably for the bee colony, fresh royal jelly contains numerous steroids and hormones, including sex and growth hormones. Because these hormones promote the growth and maturation of insect larvae, they have only limited activity in mammals.

Other important constituents of royal jelly include the following:

- Collagen, the major protein in human connective tissue, found in skin, hair, nails, bone, cartilage, tendons, ligaments, and the walls of veins and arteries
- Enzymes, including enzymes with antioxidant functions
- Immune complexes that may confer benefits similar to immune complexes found in human plasma
- Methylparaben, a powerful antioxidant that, in synthetic form, is commonly added to products as a preservative
- The nucleic acids DNA and RNA—the basic genetic building blocks of all organisms

Royal jelly can be standardized by its content of the short-chain fatty acid trans-10-hydroxy-2-decenoic acid (HDA). Fresh liquid royal jelly contains 2.0 to 6.4 percent HDA by weight. If HDA levels in a royal jelly sample are low or undetectable, it's likely that the sample has been adulterated or damaged during processing. Reputable suppliers list the HDA content of their royal jelly because it's a good indicator of a quality product.

Royal Jelly for Skin

For centuries, royal jelly has been applied to the skin to soften it, remove wrinkles, and heal eczema and dermatitis. Scientific research backs up these uses, indicating that concentrated royal jelly can improve the appearance of skin and treat various skin conditions. When fed to mice, royal jelly suppressed the development of allergic dermatitis skin lesions. In a small human study, diabetic foot ulcers healed when royal jelly was applied directly to the wounds daily for six weeks.

Collagen is the major protein in our skin. Royal jelly contains water-soluble collagen, which can be absorbed and used directly by skin cells. Soluble collagen is used in many cosmetic preparations to help rejuvenate aging and damaged skin and to smooth wrinkles. Additionally, royal jelly contains the antioxidant vitamins A, C, and E and various carotenoids that can also be absorbed by the skin. They are synergistic with collagen, acting to protect skin proteins from damage caused by exposure to sun and chemicals. People who have higher levels of skin antioxidants—especially carotenoids—have smoother, moister skin with fewer wrinkles and a reduced risk of skin cancer.

Royal jelly contains water-soluble collagen, which can be absorbed and used directly by skin cells, helping to rejuvenate aging and damaged skin. Add royal jelly to any skin lotion to amp up the benefits.

As mentioned above, royal jelly contains the hydroxy fatty acid HDA, which increases the skin's natural production of collagen. The more HDA skin cells are exposed to, the greater the collagen production.

Hydroxy fatty acids also protect the skin from dehydration and are strongly anti-inflammatory. Because of their chemical structure, these compounds help the skin retain moisture as well as help it to prevent moisture from evaporating. HDA from royal jelly blends with and fortifies the skin's natural hydroxy fatty acids, such as those derived from the essential fatty acid gamma-linolenic acid.

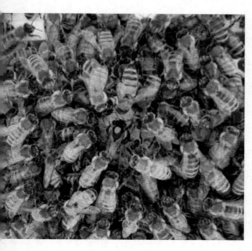

HDA probably exerts its anti-inflammatory and antiallergenic effects by working in concert with other compounds in royal jelly, particularly proteins, carotenoids, and flavonoids. Royal jelly can provide these benefits via either topical application or ingestion. HDA also has an antimicrobial effect on skin. The structure of this fatty acid is similar to that of a detergent, and to some degree this allows it to disrupt the structure of bacterial cell membranes.

Although some cosmetic and skin care products contain royal jelly, it is just one component and is usually present in only minor amounts. Such products cannot be expected to provide the benefits of pure royal jelly. To make your own skin treatments using royal jelly, see the recipes on pages 59 and 60.

Royal Jelly for Infection and Improved Immunity

One function of the mother's milk that humans and other mammals produce is to help initiate normal immune responses in the newborn. Royal jelly also plays this role. However, it is designed for bee larvae, and the overwhelming majority of honeybees live less than two months, so the immune protection bee larvae need as *individuals* is rudimentary compared to that needed by human infants and most mammals.

That said, protection of larvae is crucial to survival of the colony. Pathogens that prevent normal larval development will destroy the colony. This is so urgent that certain nurse bees spend their entire lives continually tending larvae. They are also devoted to replacing the queen should the need arise. Of course, the queen in particular must be protected from infection and premature aging. Feeding royal jelly, whether for three days or a lifetime, evidently plays a role in the colony's collective immunity.

Unique proteins isolated from royal jelly are part of the honeybee's defense system against bacterial and fungal infections. Some—including apisimin, apisin, jelleines I to IV, royalisin, and royalactin (the protein that extends the queen's life span)—are also efficacious in mammals. These compounds are effective at several hundred milligram doses, just like pharmaceutical drugs.

Apisin, a glycoprotein (a protein linked to a sugar), is of particular interest. In laboratory studies, it maintained the viability of rat liver cells for twenty days in culture and stimulated the growth of human immune cells. In both cases, this was accomplished without adding the normal cell growth medium. The glycoprotein structure may play a role in apisin's immune-boosting properties. Bacterial cell walls are made of glycoproteins, and sometimes glycoproteins from other sources can stimulate immunity as the body mistakes them for evidence of invading bacteria and mounts a protective response. This is also thought to be the reason why medicinal mushroom extracts stimulate immunity: mushrooms are fungi, and fungal cell walls are made of glycoproteins.

During an influenza epidemic in Sarajevo, Yugoslavia, it was reported that only 9 percent of patients given royal jelly daily developed the illness, compared to 40 percent of untreated patients. Unfortunately, the dose wasn't specified. However, this preventive effect may be due at least partially to royal jelly's immune-stimulating properties.

Royal jelly also has direct antimicrobial properties. One part third-day royal jelly in twenty parts water has been shown to kill several types of bacteria, including *E. coli*, after three hours of exposure. This effect was heightened by mixing the royal jelly with honey. Royal jelly collected from three-day-old larvae has the highest quality and also the most powerful antimicrobial activity. Luckily, royal jelly is also most abundant on the third day.

Royal Jelly for Lowering Cholesterol and Triglycerides

A variety of studies have shown that royal jelly can help lower levels of cholesterol and triglycerides. In human studies, consuming 50 to 100 milligrams of freeze-dried royal jelly per day decreased total serum cholesterol by 14 percent and triglycerides by 10 percent, an effect also seen in animal studies. Royal jelly supplementation also slowed the development of atherosclerosis in rabbits fed high-fat diets.

Chinese researchers found that freeze-dried royal jelly lowered total cholesterol but increased HDL (good cholesterol) in rats with high cholesterol and triglyceride levels. The dosage was 700 milligrams per kilogram of body weight per day for six weeks. This treatment also lowered the risk of developing clots in the bloodstream, which lead to heart attack, stroke, and phlebitis. However, extrapolating the amounts in this study to a human scale indicates that a 70-kilogram (155-pound) human would need to consume about 50 grams of freeze-dried royal jelly daily, or 150 grams of fresh—clearly an excessive dose.

HDA isolated from royal jelly was found to be particularly effective in conferring these benefits. I hypothesize that HDA, being a hydroxy fatty acid, has actions similar to those of 13-hydroxyoctadecadienoic acid (13-HODE), a hydroxy fatty acid metabolized from linoleic acid. Present in normal artery walls, 13-HODE inhibits atherosclerosis and blood clot damage.

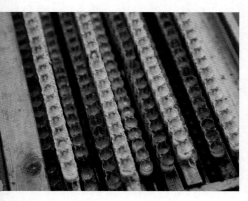

As mentioned, royal jelly contains all the B vitamins and is especially rich in pantothenic acid. It also contains acetylcholine, phosphatidylcholine, phytosterols (mainly beta-sitosterol), and insect steroid hormones that mimic estrogen and testosterone. All of these compounds help lower cholesterol, and if you could eat enough royal jelly, it might make you feel younger.

While some people claim that taking very small doses, such as 100 milligrams of fresh royal jelly daily, can yield benefits, this hasn't stood up in controlled research. A realistic dosage for significant health improvements in an adult with cardiovascular disease is 3 to 7 grams of fresh royal jelly per day.

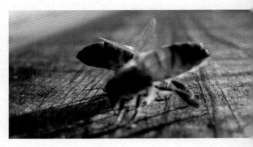

Royal Jelly for Lowering Blood Pressure

In rat studies, royal jelly has safely and effectively lowered blood pressure, and anecdotal evidence indicates it may have the same effects in humans. It doesn't have this activity until it is digested and its proteins are broken down into peptides, short chains of two to about ten amino acids linked together. Certain peptides have biological activities, including acting as enzymes.

Some of the peptides from royal jelly have the ability to block the enzyme that makes angiotensin, a naturally occurring hormone that acts to constrict blood vessels and therefore raises blood pressure. You may have heard of ACE inhibitors (angiotensin-converting-enzyme inhibitors), a common type of blood pressure medication. Peptides from royal jelly can work like ACE inhibitors.

Purchasing and Storing Royal Jelly

The highest-quality royal jelly products usually come from manufacturers with a full line of bee products. Because royal jelly is exceedingly fragile and perishable and damaged by exposure to heat or light, professional apicultural, processing, and distribution practices are needed to ensure the integrity of the product.

Royal jelly is available commercially in fresh and freeze-dried form. Fresh royal jelly can be purchased as a liquid or as soft-gel capsules. Both should be stored in the refrigerator, and there should be an expiration date on the bottle. Don't purchase vials of royal jelly that have been stored at room temperature for an indeterminate period. I also recommend against vials imported from Asian countries, as these are typically undated, poorly marked, and have no manufacturer listed, so there is no one you can contact if you don't like the product or have questions.

Fresh royal jelly is often sold mixed with honey, which acts as a natural preservative for the royal jelly and protects it well if the product is stored tightly capped and out of direct heat and light. After the container is opened, it can be stored at room temperature for several months. However, if you don't use it up quickly or your home is warm, it's best to refrigerate it.

Royal jelly can be successfully freeze-dried, which keeps it fresh, viable, and stable at room temperature. It also has the advantage of being concentrated. Freeze-dried royal jelly is sold in capsule and tablet form.

Using Royal Jelly

Sample only a tiny amount of royal jelly initially in case you're allergic to it. As with all bee products, be especially cautious if you're allergic to bee stings. If you have no adverse reaction, there's no risk in taking 10 to 20 grams of fresh, liquid royal jelly per day to help heal a medical condition. If taking it preventively, 1 to 2 grams is a good daily dose. You can double or triple this dose if you are elderly, have an impaired immune system, or are recovering from illness or injury. If you prefer to use the freeze-dried form, 1 gram of liquid royal jelly is equivalent to 200 to 300 milligrams of freeze-dried—typically the amount in 1 capsule or tablet.

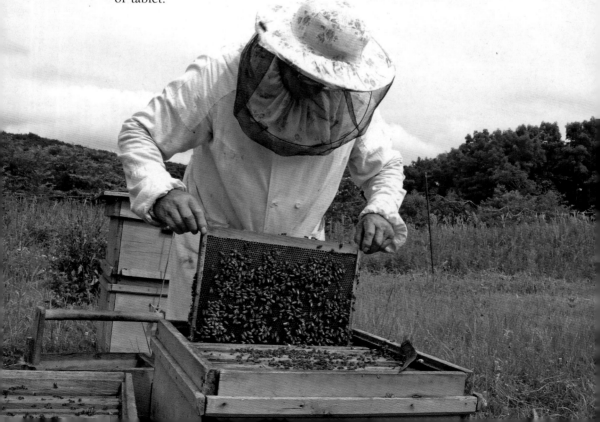

HONEY

Honey is made from flower nectar collected by worker bees in spring, summer, and early autumn. Some worker bees also collect the sugary secretions of aphids that feed on tree sap, a substance known as honeydew. The gathered nectar is stored in wax cells, thousands of which form the honeycomb. It is concentrated as the bees fan the comb with their wings to drive off excess moisture. In a natural honeybee colony, honey serves as food for the bees through the winter, when plants are dormant. In an apiculture hive, most of the honeycomb is removed to harvest the honey and beeswax, and the beekeeper provides sugar or corn syrup solution to sustain the bees.

Beekeepers earn most of their income by renting bee colonies to farmers and orchardists. The hives are transported to places where important crops are blooming, and the bees pollinate the crops as they gather nectar and pollen. Pollinating California's almond trees alone requires about one million bee colonies. The tasty result of all this pollination effort is honey. Global honey production is worth over $1.25 billion annually. While that's a significant amount, it's only a fraction of the value of the bees' pollination efforts, which are estimated to be worth $16 billion annually to agriculture in the United States alone.

For millennia, honey has been appreciated for its delicious sweet flavor and digestibility. In both ancient and modern times, Buddhist, Christian, Hindu, Moslem, and Native American cultures have revered the honeybee. China has a continuous tradition of apiculture that stretches back over three thousand years. In the 1600s, workers in Shenyang collected 2,500 to 3,000 kilograms of honey each year just to supply the Manchu Imperial Palace. Globally, it wasn't until after the Industrial Revolution that sugar became more widely available than honey. In preindustrial times, Europeans ate about as much honey as they do sugar today—15 to 30 kilograms per year.

Honey is 15 to 21 percent water by weight, with almost all of the remainder consisting of carbohydrate. About 85 percent of the solids in honey are the simple sugars glucose and fructose. Also included are minor amounts of sucrose, maltose, and other sugars, the exact com-

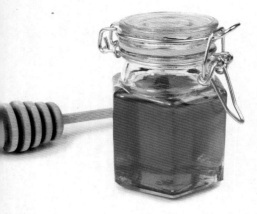

position varying with the honey. In addition, honey contains larger, complex sugar molecules called oligosaccharides. Although we humans can't easily digest oligosaccharides, the beneficial bacteria in our guts thrive on them, so they are valuable prebiotics. (Prebiotics are nondigestible components of food that promote the growth of beneficial microorganisms in the intestines.) As I'll discuss later, moderate amounts of honey can be beneficial for diabetes, and its oligosaccharide content is one of the reasons for this.

The sugar molecules in honey are strongly attracted to its water and bond to it. This is one reason why honey is a viscous syrup, not a crystalline solid like table sugar (pure sucrose). When honey is dried, it rapidly reabsorbs water from the atmosphere and returns to its liquid state. However, honey does crystallize sometimes. This can occur spontaneously in a jar that has been on the shelf for a while, or it may be purposely crystallized to make spreadable honey products. However, even when crystallized, honey is still sticky and contains lots of water.

Honey: A Botanical Product

Less than 4 percent of honey consists of phytochemicals from the plants that supplied the nectar, but this minor fraction is responsible for the endless variations in honey. Unprocessed or lightly processed honey retains the flavor and aroma of the nectar source plants, making it truly special. In fact, high-quality unprocessed honey is like fine wine, with the source plants, growing location, season, climate, weather, processing, and just plain luck influencing the color, aroma, and flavor. Commercial beehives placed in orange groves produce fragrant orange-scented honey, while those in white clover fields produce light, mild, all-purpose honey. Nectar from buckwheat flowers yields strong, dark, musky honey that's an excellent substitute for molasses in baking or barbecue sauce. However, buckwheat honey is like buckwheat pancakes—definitely an acquired taste for many people.

The various and numerous phytochemicals in honey not only influence the honey's flavor and aroma but also have antioxidant and healing properties and provide nutritional benefits.

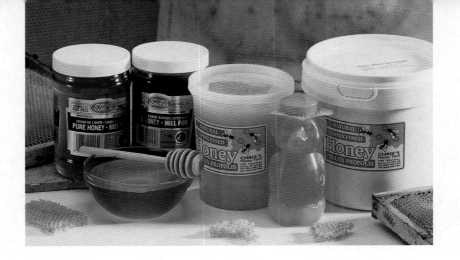

The various phytochemicals in honey not only influence the honey's flavor and aroma but also have antioxidant and healing properties and provide nutritional benefits. Apicultural scientists are interested in identifying the phytochemical composition of honey for several reasons. Most importantly, the trace phytochemicals in honey provide a fingerprint that can be used to identify the source plants visited by the bees. Phytochemicals in honey are extracted and then compared to phytochemical extracts and pollen from likely source plants near the hives where the honey originated.

In any given foraging area, many potential source plants exist and may be represented in the honey. But in practice, bees repeatedly visit favorite plants, presumably because these plants provide more abundant and nutritious nectar and pollen. These plants may also be more accessible or attractive to bees. Less competition from other insects is another factor. Identifying preferred source plants yields information on which plants keep bees healthy and productive and helps beekeepers know where to place their hives.

There are also some source plants that beekeepers don't want their bees to visit. For example, wild tropical honeys occasionally poison animals because the flowers of the source plants are poisonous to mammals but not to insects. Honey with a high concentration of nectar from certain plants in the heath family, including mountain laurel, sheep laurel, and some species of rhododendron, can contain poisonous compounds called grayanotoxins, which can cause nausea, vomiting, excessive

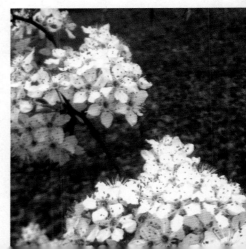

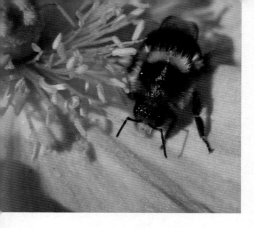

perspiration, and dizziness. If the honey is eaten only in moderation, these symptoms will resolve with no permanent effects once the honey is no longer consumed. However, the poisoning can be life-threatening if these honeys are eaten in large quantities. That said, most cases of grayanotoxin poisoning have occurred when children, livestock, or pets consumed the source plants, not honey derived from them.

Phytochemical fingerprinting is also useful for legal reasons. For honey to be labeled as unifloral (from a single floral source), 51 percent of its nectar or 45 percent of its traces of pollen must be from the designated source plant. Although these percentages seem low (can you imagine orange juice that's required to be only 51 percent from oranges?), there's no practical way to further control the content. So even when hives are located in the middle of a vast clover field, for example, laboratory identification of characteristic clover phytochemicals or pollen is required in order for the honey to be labeled and sold as "clover honey."

Over time, characteristic phytochemical patterns in popular honey varieties began to emerge, and it was not lost on researchers that many of the phytochemicals in those fingerprints are active ingredients in herbal preparations. For example, Australian eucalyptus honeys are identified by small amounts of eucalyptus essential oil components (including cineole and menthol) and the flavonoids myricetin, kaempferol, luteolin, and tricetin. Orange-blossom honey has a small amount of orange essential oil (including citral and limonene) and the flavonoid hesperetin. Malaysian honey, with nectar from *Melaleuca cajuputi* (gelam tree), a cousin of the tea tree (*Melaleuca alternifolia*), is a source of cajeput, which is similar to tea tree oil. Likewise, honeys from heather, rosemary, sage, and thyme have small amounts of the essential oils characteristic of those plants, resulting in distinctive aromas and flavors in the honey and also contributing medicinal benefits.

Antioxidants in Honey

Floral honeys can contain relatively high levels of phytochemical antioxidants from the source plants. The highest reported antioxidant content in a unifloral US commercial honey was in Illinois buckwheat honey, and the lowest was in California sage honey, with the buckwheat honey being twenty times richer in antioxidants than the sage honey. Other US honeys with high antioxidant content include Hawaiian Christmas berry, sunflower, and water tupelo. Among Canadian varieties, blueberry, buckwheat, and tupelo honeys are highest in antioxidant capacity. European winners include fir, hawthorn, mixed forest, pine, raspberry, and thyme.

All studies concur that the darker the honey, the higher the antioxidant content. Although lighter, transparent honeys, such as clover, lime, mesquite, and orange are more common, they are less remarkable in their antioxidant content. In contrast, buckwheat, eucalyptus, fir, pine, and water tupelo are dark brown or greenish brown and translucent. When humans ingest dark honeys, their bloodstream antioxidant capacity reliably increases.

The major antioxidant phytochemicals in honey are identical to those in fruits, vegetables, herbal products, bee pollen, and propolis. Most important are flavonoids and other phenolic compounds. Darker honeys are dark precisely because they have higher concentrations of phenolics, which impart brown, green, or dark yellow colors. This higher phenolic content accounts for most of the increased antioxidant activity. Ascorbic acid (vitamin C) and other organic acids (caffeic, cinnamic, gluconic, hydroxybenzoic, and malic) are other important antioxidants in honey.

Although honeybees are native to Europe, they easily adapt to new types of vegetation, creating variations not just in the honey produced but also in the pollen collected, propolis, and royal jelly. A key determinant of the phenolic and flavonoid content of honeys is whether they are from temperate or tropical regions. Just as fruits from temperate and tropical locales differ in terms of flavor, aroma, and texture, so do honeys. Major antioxidant flavonoids found in all temperate-climate honeys studied are chrysin, galangin, pinobanksin, and pinocembrin.

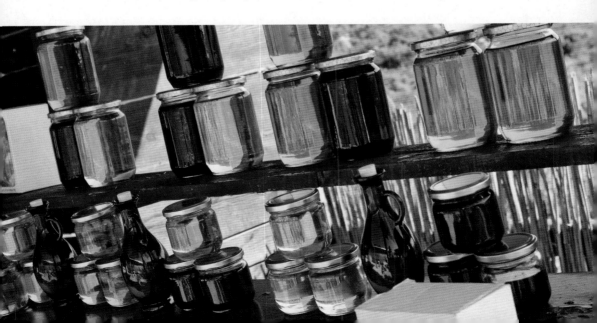

Honeys from the southern hemisphere have their own distinctive compositions. Some that are exceptionally rich in antioxidants include those sourced from Malaysian gelam trees, New Zealand manuka trees, and, in Australia, various trees in the genus *Eucalyptus* (red river gum, mallee, and yellow box).

Honey as Part of a Nutritious Diet

Honey, especially raw honey, is nutritionally superior to white, brown, and "raw" sugars and fructose. Its sugars are easily digested, and the vitamins, minerals, and enzymes present in raw honey aid digestion and metabolism. Prebiotic oligosaccharides provide another nutritional boost, allowing honey to act as a soluble fiber.

The natural antioxidants and essential oils in honey act as preservatives. Honey can even serve as a safe, natural preservative for other foods, including sliced deli meats, sausage, and ground meats.

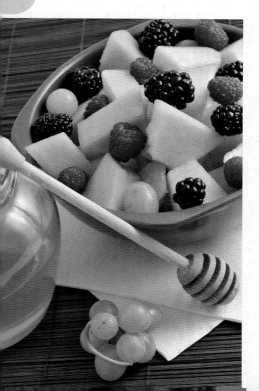

Honey has a long shelf life compared to a sugar solution of similar concentration and viscosity. One reason is that its natural antioxidants and essential oils act as preservatives. In fact, honey can serve as a safe, natural preservative for other foods, with buckwheat, soybean, and tupelo honeys being among the best choices for this purpose.

Dipping fresh-cut fruits such as apples and pears into honey slows browning due to oxidation. Likewise, stirring a bit of honey and $1/8$ to $1/4$ teaspoon of vitamin C powder into a fruit salad will keep it fresh longer while also improving its nutritional value.

Most people use honey in tea or coffee or on toast, waffles, or pancakes. You can also use it as a sweetener when making barbecue sauces, salad dressings, vegetable dips, lemonade, and iced tea. It's best to use it in unheated preparations or to add it after heating, as the natural vitamin C and most of the other antioxidant organic acids are destroyed by heat.

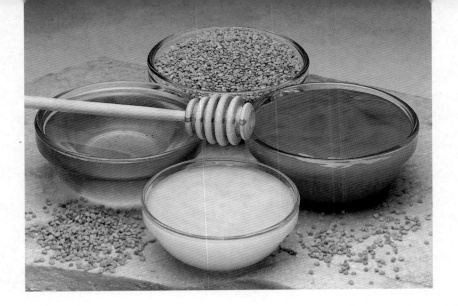

Honey, Diabetes, and Metabolic Syndrome

Although honey is superior to sugar, in comparison to fruits and vegetables it is lower in phytochemicals and much higher in sugar. Therefore, it's a good substitute for refined sugar, but it shouldn't replace fruits, vegetables, or herbal preparations. Remember, about 85 percent of honey consists of glucose and fructose, so it's a highly concentrated source of simple sugars. Excessive consumption is particularly contraindicated for anyone with diabetes, abnormal glucose tolerance, hypertension, or obesity. However, when used in modest amounts as a sweetener, honey can benefit diabetics and can even aid in weight loss.

Because honey contains a great deal of fructose, you may wonder how it can possibly be healthful, given the growing concern about high-fructose corn syrup (HFCS). To adequately address this complex topic, I must first provide a bit of information about HFCS and its downsides. In the United States, consumption of this highly processed sweetener increased by more than 1,000 percent between 1970 and 1990, far exceeding changes in intake of any other food or food group. HFCS now accounts for more than 40 percent of caloric sweeteners added to foods and beverages.

It hasn't escaped notice that increased use of HFCS in the United States has mirrored rapid increases in obesity and type 2 diabetes. However, only when people drink a lot of sodas and sweetened juices and teas—consuming on the order of 100 grams of fructose per day—is there a strong link between HFCS and obesity and metabolic syndrome. (Metabolic syndrome, a condition that greatly increases the risk of cancer, cardiovascular disease, chronic inflammation, and type 2 diabetes, is a complex disorder that involves many factors, including genetics, diet, and environmental conditions. However, the primary cause is obesity.) Additionally, high consumption of soft drinks is correlated with high intakes of fast foods, chips, candy, and baked goods, which are definitely linked to obesity and metabolic syndrome.

Honey, particularly darker varieties, contains numerous powerful antioxidants, including some that are nonexistent or rare in fruits and vegetables.

Modest amounts of fructose contained in fruits, vegetables, and honey have always been part of the human diet and are beneficial. In every human and animal study to date, consuming honey has proven to be beneficial or neutral with respect to controlling blood sugar, never harmful. However, the current consumption of large amounts of fructose in refined foods is unprecedented. Human metabolism isn't equipped to deal with this excess, particularly in the form of HFCS, which didn't even exist before the mid-1900s.

In contrast to HFCS, in moderate amounts honey confers the following potential benefits that may not only help to improve overall health but may also mitigate symptoms of diabetes and metabolic syndrome:

- Honey's natural blend of sugars are released into the bloodstream more slowly than sucrose, so honey doesn't spike blood sugar levels as much as sugar and HFCS.
- The prebiotic oligosaccharides in honey are helpful in promoting good digestion and regulating blood sugar levels.
- Honey provides a stronger feeling of satiety than refined sugars.
- Honey doesn't raise levels of triglycerides or LDL (bad cholesterol) or increase blood pressure.
- Honey, particularly darker varieties, contains numerous powerful antioxidants, including some that are nonexistent or rare in fruits and vegetables.

I believe that metabolic syndrome is not a disease; rather, it is the predictable response of human physiology, evolved over eons, to chronic "high-calorie malnutrition." By that, I mean heavy consumption of refined and processed foods that don't contain enough vitamins, trace elements, and fiber to metabolize the calories in the food. Honey has the advantage of being a natural food that human physiology is adapted to, and consequently it isn't implicated in blood sugar problems and can instead be part of the solution.

Honey: A Natural Antibiotic and Antiseptic

In ancient times, honey was revered for its healing properties. Greek, Roman, Islamic, Chinese, Egyptian, sub-Saharan, and Native American cultures all used honey medicinally. It has been utilized to treat colds, diarrhea, flus, indigestion, skin and stomach ulcers, sore throats, and wounds. Research has strongly confirmed the healing properties of honey—more definitively than for any other natural product. Raw unprocessed honey is a broad-spectrum antibiotic, inhibiting the growth of numerous pathogenic bacteria. Even when highly diluted, honey has antimicrobial properties. Some honeys are effective against skin fungi as well.

Honey may prove to be especially beneficial in fighting antibiotic-resistant infections in hospitals and clinics, which have become so common that some surgical patients must be quarantined. Most of these infections are from staphylococcus bacteria, which are often naturally present on the skin. If you have a large wound or surgical incision and skin bacteria in the area can't be controlled, you're at tremendous risk for a disfiguring scar or even a life-threatening infection.

Because honey is known to kill bacteria cultured from septic wounds, it has been investigated for its ability to treat infections resistant to standard antibiotics, particularly by noted honey researcher Peter Molan at the University of Waikato, New Zealand. In over one hundred reports describing thousands of different patients, his team found that honey cleared up infections that were unresponsive to conventional antiseptics and antibiotics. It quickly healed wounds that were infected with dangerous strains of staphylococcus resistant to penicillin or multiple antibiotics. Molan and his colleagues cultured *Staphylococcus aureus* and various species of pseudomonas bacteria collected directly from infected patient wounds and, based on their studies, concluded that honey dressings could prevent the growth of these bacteria in wounds, even when diluted as much as fourteenfold by body fluids. However, if dressings are changed several times per day, the honey should never

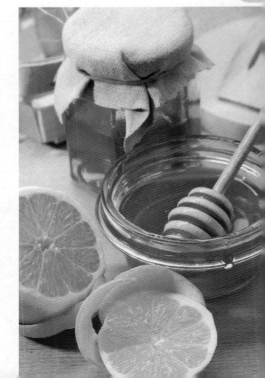

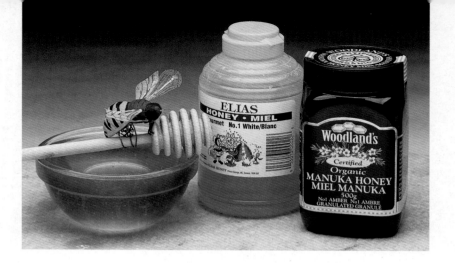

become this diluted. Manuka honey was the most effective of fifty-eight honeys tested against *Staphylococcus aureus* and maintained its ability to kill this pathogen even when diluted by a factor of fifty-six. It was also far more effective against pseudomonas than mixed-pasture honey was.

Brazilian researchers have found tropical South American honeys to be similarly effective against *Staphylococcus aureus*, and Canadian researchers found blueberry and buckwheat honeys effective against *E. coli*. Malaysian tualang honey is especially effective against several types of bacteria that infect people who have serious burns and compromised immune systems.

Overall, antimicrobial activity is generally higher in stronger-tasting honeys from aromatic plants such as conifers, culinary herbs, eucalyptus, mint, and species in the genus *Melaleuca*. And as with antioxidant activity, antimicrobial activity also tends to be stronger in darker honeys.

New Zealand's manuka honey, mentioned above in conjunction with Peter Molan's research, is considered superior for medicinal use. Overall, manuka honey, sold under the brand name Medihoney, is effective against more types of bacteria at lower doses than any other honey known. This stands to reason, given that essential oil extracted from the manuka tree has long been used topically to prevent or cure fungal and bacterial infections and soothe diaper rash, dermatitis, and psoriasis. It has also been used in mouthwashes and rinses to kill oral bacteria.

The effective antimicrobial properties of manuka essential oil are derived in part from the terpenoids cineol, cymene, myrcene, and pinene, which are also present in the dark, fragrant honey. In addition, manuka honey has a high total concentration of phenolics and other flavonoids and a notably wide variety of phytochemicals in general, some of which have not been found in other honeys. Some of them, such as caffeic acid and methylglyoxal, are powerful antimicrobial agents. Finally, manuka honey has a relatively high protein content, which causes the honey to set up like a gel, making wound dressing easier and less messy.

Honey for Wounds and Skin Infections

Ancient warriors carried raw honey with them to treat battlefield wounds, as it was known that cuts, abrasions, or burns covered with a layer of honey would heal more rapidly and with less chance of infection. Raw honey mixed with propolis was also utilized in this way.

Honey has been used successfully to heal many types of lingering or chronic skin infections or wounds, including abscesses, bedsores, boils, burns, cuts, gangrene, skin grafts, surgical incisions, and various sorts of skin ulcers. It's equally effective for animals, healing wounds resulting from a variety of causes, including veterinary surgery. Here is a summary of some of the properties that give honey its amazing wound-healing power:

- Honey reduces infection, inflammation, weeping, and foul odors.
- Honey heals wounds faster and more cleanly than other treatments.
- Honey actively promotes the growth of healthy new skin.
- Honey doesn't cause dermatitis or allergic reactions.
- Honey dressings soothe pain and itching.
- Honey dressings soften scabs and gently remove crusts and dead tissue.

Honey has been used to treat tough medical cases that weren't responding to conventional treatment, such as diabetic ulcers that had festered for one to three years. What a welcome relief that must be for patients suffering from such challenging health issues. Honey is also a gentler, far more tolerable agent for removing dead tissue from sore, infected wounds, whereas surgical removal (debridement) is exceedingly painful. Patients whose wounds are literally untouchable are able to have their wounds properly cleaned when honey dressings are used.

Studies have shown that honey-impregnated gauze is better than or at least the equivalent of its conventional counterparts in preventing infection in burns and varicose ulcers. It also has proved to promote faster and more effective healing than conventional treatments, including hydrofiber silver gels, hydrogels, gauze infused with silver sulfadiazine (an antiseptic), polyurethane film, and amniotic membrane. Plus, amniotic membrane is a very expensive and specialized dressing, especially compared to honey and gauze.

Wound infections following cesarean section or hysterectomy healed faster and more cleanly with honey than the standard alcohol-and-iodine treatment. Honey treatments reduced the average postoperative scar width by nearly two-thirds and the duration of hospitalization by half.

Mutya Subrahmanyam, MD, a specialist in burn treatment, has reported that skin grafts can be stored in honey at room temperature. After six weeks of storage, there was a 100 percent success rate for graft uptake, and after twelve weeks the success rate was 80 percent. In addition, treating wounds with honey prior to skin grafting operations resulted in better graft uptake. Finally, the large stripping-type wounds at skin graft donor sites healed faster and with less pain when dressed with honey-impregnated gauzes than with paraffin gauzes or saline-soaked gauzes. When compared to hydrocolloid, an expensive specialized wound dressing, healing was essentially the same but much less costly. In all of these cases honey saved both the hospital and patients considerable time and expense. Given that honey is so effective, safe, affordable, and practical for skin graft surgery, you can see what a great option it is for your minor cuts and abrasions!

Honey for Dermatitis, Hemorrhoids, and Fungal Infections of the Skin

Saudi physician Noori Al-Waili, an expert on medicinal honey, has successfully treated many patients with skin fungal infections, diaper rash, hemorrhoids, and anal fissures with a salve made of equal parts honey, olive oil, and beeswax. This salve is an ancient treatment mentioned in the Bible and Koran. He also used the salve for allergic dermatitis and psoriasis, and within two weeks, more than half of the patients who received this treatment had skin that was softer and less red and itchy. In addition, all of these patients reduced their use of steroid drugs by 75 percent without experiencing flare-ups. Once again, honey treatments cost less and also had no side effects compared to standard drug therapy.

Honey for Gastric and Oral Healing

Honey was a remedy for indigestion, ulcers, diarrhea, and various stomach pains throughout the ancient world, thanks to its antimicrobial and healing properties. Case reports from New Zealand physicians especially recommend manuka honey for gastric healing and protection. A combination of bee products can also be effective. For example, taking a mixture of honey, royal jelly, and propolis on an empty stomach fifteen minutes before bedtime may heal stomach ulcers and prevent heartburn (see page 62 for specific information on using this remedy).

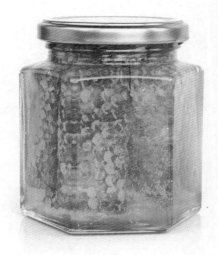

Honey is effective against pediatric infectious gastroenteritis, which causes diarrhea, vomiting, and fever and is a major problem worldwide. In one study, 196 infants and children with gastroenteritis were assigned to receive either 5 percent glucose (the standard treatment) or 5 percent honey in a rehydration solution. All who received honey recovered as well as or better than those who received glucose. A subgroup diagnosed with bacterial infections recovered in an average time of fifty-eight hours when given honey, compared to ninety-three hours with glucose.

Acids produced by oral bacteria are responsible for eroding dental enamel and eventually causing cavities. Perhaps surprisingly, given honey's sugar content, it may help fight tooth decay. In a study that compared a chewable "honey leather" made with manuka honey to sugarless gum for the control group, thirty subjects chewed or sucked either the honey product or gum for ten minutes, three times a day, after each meal. The honey product was found to be twice as effective as sugarless gum in reducing plaque levels and gum bleeding. The antibacterial effect of manuka honey was so strong that it overrode the potential detrimental effect of the sugars in the honey.

Persistent mouth sores (mucositis) are a side effect of radiation treatment for cancer, and conventional medicine offers no effective remedy for this condition. However, patients with mucositis who were given honey daily after radiation had fewer sores, less pain, and fewer oral infections compared to those who received standard care, which in this case essentially means doing nothing. Honey made it possible for one-third of patients to eat properly during radiation therapy. Mucositis may respond even better to honey mixed with royal jelly and propolis.

How Honey Heals Wounds

All raw honey contains propolis and bee pollen, which have healing properties outlined in earlier chapters. In addition to these, there are five major properties of honey that make it such a powerful agent for healing wounds.

HYDROPHILIC SUGARS. All honey is 15 to 21 percent water. Most of the remainder is glucose and fructose. These sugars are strongly attracted to the water and bond to it to form a syrup. This property is valuable because a layer of honey over a wound will absorb fluids from the wound, desiccating bacteria and fungi and inhibiting their growth. This is the primary reason why honey rapidly clears wound infections.

GLUCOSE OXIDASE. Raw honey contains the enzyme glucose oxidase, which breaks down glucose, producing hydrogen peroxide in the process. This only occurs when the honey comes into contact with water or water-rich fluids. When raw honey comes into contact with body fluids leaking from an open wound, the enzyme is activated. Hydrogen peroxide is a powerful antiseptic and anti-inflammatory. While fine for initial sterilization, it irritates tissues and prevents healing when continually used on wounds. However, the glucose oxidase in honey produces small but steady amounts of hydrogen peroxide—just enough to sterilize wounds and stimulate tissue repair but not so much that it interferes with healing. Once the wound heals and dries up, the glucose oxidase is no longer activated, so no unneeded peroxide is produced. Keep in mind that the naturally occurring enzymes in honey are destroyed by pasteurizing and heating, improper storage, and bright light, so most commercial honeys lack the ability to make hydrogen peroxide.

COMPLEX COMPOSITION. Floral honey contains additional healing and antiseptic compounds, with the composition varying depending on the plants from which the honey originated. Stronger, darker honeys and those derived from aromatic plants have greater antioxidant and antimicrobial activity. For medicinal use, honeys derived from buckwheat, eucalyptus, manuka, sage, thyme, or mixed desert plants are good, readily available choices. In India, neem and lotus honeys are revered for their healing properties, as are gelam and tualang honeys in Malaysia.

ANTI-INFLAMMATORY PROPERTIES. Honey is anti-inflammatory. Wounds that aren't healing well are almost always afflicted with chronic inflammation. This often manifests as a ring of angry red tissue doming up around a wound. Inflamed wounds cause pain, burning, and itching.

ACIDITY. Honey is naturally acidic, with a pH in the range of 3.2 to 4.5, which inhibits the growth of many microorganisms. This is a major reason why honey keeps so well on the shelf. Note that when honey is diluted, its acidity decreases. When honey is used on an open wound, it's constantly in contact with body fluids, which dilute the honey, rendering it less acidic. Therefore, the acidic antimicrobial action of honey is not sustained and can only partially account for honey's healing effects.

Purchasing and Storing Honey

Despite its medicinal properties, honey is purchased primarily for its flavor. Raw honey that's unprocessed or only lightly processed retains the flavors and aromas of the nectar source plants, but its characteristics can vary widely. Highly processed honey has a more predictable flavor, but it's also bland and unexceptional. Medicinally and nutritionally, raw honey is the best choice. It is extracted from the comb with a minimum of processing and isn't overheated or sterilized. It contains active enzymes, vitamins, and volatile chemical constituents that are destroyed or removed by heating and processing. If you have children, start giving them raw honey early (but not until they are ten to twelve months old) so their palates become educated to flavors beyond just sweet.

To find flavorful, high-quality honeys, visit a farmers' market or natural food store in an area known for apiculture. Specialty markets, particularly those with goods from Russia, the Baltic states, eastern Europe, the Middle East, Korea, or Japan often have an extensive selection of beehive products. You may want to purchase strong, dark, aromatic honeys for medicinal use and lighter honeys for table use.

After opening, honey can be stored in a sealed container at room temperature, out of direct heat and light, for at least four months and usually six. For longer storage, or if your home is warm, keep a small jar at room temperature and refrigerate the remainder until needed. If

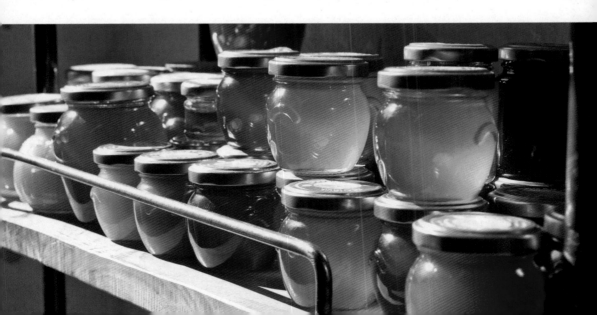

honey crystallizes, heat it in the microwave in a microwave-safe container for five to fifteen seconds on high power; the crystals will readily melt. You can also put the whole container, tightly sealed, in a hot water bath to reliquefy the honey.

Precautions for Using Honey

Raw, unprocessed honey can cause allergic reactions due to the presence of small amounts of certain phytochemicals, pollen, or bee dander. Sometimes switching to another variety of honey or using processed honey solves the problem.

Children under ten to twelve months of age should not be fed raw or pasteurized honey unless under medical supervision. Although honey is relatively sterile, it may contain some hardy bacterial and fungal spores that can survive pasteurization. While the minor amount of spores in honey poses no risk for adults or even toddlers, infants may suffer serious infections, particularly botulism.

Botulism is caused by a virulent toxin produced by the bacterium *Clostridium botulinum*, which naturally exists in soils. The bacterial spores don't germinate inside adult humans or children because our stomach acid kills them. However, because infants don't produce strong stomach acid, the spores can germinate in their intestines. Honey used topically to treat minor wounds and infections doesn't pose a botulism risk unless it can be licked off. (Note that it wouldn't make sense to heat honey to very high temperatures to render it sterile for infant consumption, as this would destroy its healing properties.)

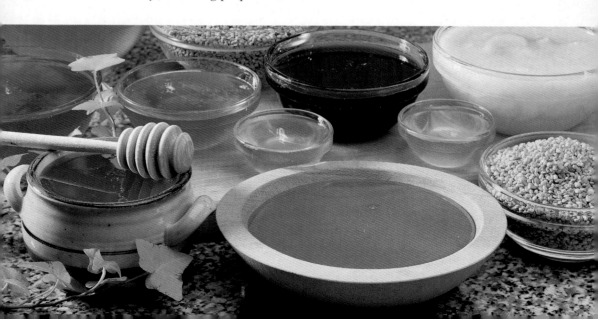

USING BEE PRODUCTS FOR HEALING

As emphasized throughout this book, bees collectively possess the largest body of knowledge of flowering plants in existence. Their expertise in botany, phytochemicals, and medicinal plants is profound, and it's abundantly reflected in the remarkable healing properties of all the beehive products. Their amassed wisdom is as valuable to us as it is to them, and it can play a crucial role in protecting both human and bee societies.

The preceding chapters offered a great deal of information about the four medicinal beehive products and what bees have to teach us. In this chapter, I'll share some information on using these products—pollen, propolis, royal jelly, and honey—medicinally. I'll begin with some general guidelines and conclude with recipes for remedies that I've developed over the years. This chapter will help you take a hands-on approach to health and healing. As you learn to use bee products medicinally and to make your own home remedies with beehive products, the results will speak for themselves. Indeed, you'll set such a compelling example that others will follow.

Making Bee Pollen Palatable

Children usually don't like to eat bee pollen by the spoonful, and the same is true of some adults. You can purchase chewable pollen wafers, but they are expensive, and picky eaters will still reject them. Unfortunately, these are exactly the people who tend to eat insufficient amounts of produce and therefore can benefit most from supplemental bee pollen.

As mentioned in the chapter on bee pollen, don't make the mistake of trying to sneak a bit of bee pollen in a large amount of food. Its distinctive flavor will be noticeable, and your cover will be blown. Instead, make up small, bite-sized morsels, as these will be far more tolerable. For children, make consumption mandatory, just like a chewable vitamin. If you opt to experiment and create your own pollen treats, just remember that pollen's nutrients are fragile. *Never put pollen directly into hot foods or bake with it.* As people's palates grow accustomed to the pollen, you can gradually increase the amount.

Here are a few recipe suggestions:

- Dip a small piece of dark chocolate in honey, then roll it in bee pollen. You can mix the bee pollen with chopped nuts or cookie crumbs. The entire morsel should be eaten at once, without licking off the coating.
- Make crispy rice cereal treats. If those eating the treats can tolerate chocolate and peanut butter, use cocoa-flavored crispy rice cereal and substitute warm peanut butter for the margarine. After spreading the mixture in a pan and allowing it to *cool completely*, cut it into small squares. To assemble each morsel, put some bee pollen on top, about $1/2$ teaspoon, and roll into a bite-sized ball.
- Mix about $1/2$ cup of peanut or almond butter with 1 cup of crispy rice cereal and 1 scant tablespoon of bee pollen. Form the mixture into bite-sized balls. If they're sticky, roll them in a bit of additional cereal. The cereal must be sweet, so you may want to use a flavored variety.

Treating Respiratory Infections

It's important to realize that you don't usually "catch" a cold or upper respiratory infection. The viruses and bacteria that cause these are already present in your body and the surrounding environment, and your immune system usually keeps them in check. However, if you've been stressed, unhappy, sleeping or eating poorly, or otherwise neglecting your health, the microbes can proliferate to a level where they cause symptoms. Fortunately, taking propolis can often help prevent illness, or if you do get sick, it can reduce the severity or duration of symptoms.

During cold and flu season, I recommend taking 500 milligrams of propolis daily as a preventive measure. When taking airline flights or tending people who are sick, increase the amount to 1,000 milligrams daily.

As soon as you feel a sore throat or sinus congestion coming on, coat your throat with propolis spray four or five times a day. Alternatively, or in addition to the propolis spray, you can take 3 capsules (a total of 1.5 grams or 1,500 milligrams) of propolis per day or 1 dropper of propolis extract four or five times a day. Also take 1,000 to 2,000 milligrams of vitamin C each time and get in bed as soon a possible. Getting twelve hours of sleep and taking these supplements will probably prevent you from developing a full-blown cold or sinus infection. If you don't feel you have the time to rest, keep this in mind: one day of resting and taking care of your health may well prevent seven days of misery and poor work performance.

You can enhance the success of this approach by adding other powerful botanical products that interfere with the growth of common respiratory pathogens and help flush them out of the body. A good combination is propolis, Japanese honeysuckle bud (*Lonicera japonica*), and forsythia berry (*Forsythia suspensa*). You can use either capsules or extracts. If using capsules, take 3 capsules of each four or five times daily with plenty of water. If using extracts, mix them together and take them all at once to minimize tasting them.

Honey can also be helpful. Two to four times a day, drink a cup of hot tea (preferably decaffeinated, so you can sleep) with 1 to 2 tablespoons of honey mixed in and one slice each of orange and lemon (with the peel) added. Sip gently to coat your throat.

If you have an existing respiratory infection, follow this protocol in conjunction with taking antibiotic drugs, not in place of them. I recommend taking 4 to 8 grams of propolis per day to help clear upper respiratory infections.

Treating Inflammation and Associated Pain

Propolis doses of 3 to 5 grams, or 3 to 5 droppers of liquid extract, per day are required to reduce pain associated with chronic inflammation. (As with all bee products, if you are allergic to bee stings, be especially cautious about using propolis.) After four to six weeks, you can reduce this dose by half if you are experiencing good results.

For treating acute inflammation (such as hay fever, insect stings, sinusitis, sports injuries, or sprains), use 4 to 7 grams or droppers per day for three to six days. Please consult a health care professional if acute inflammation continues unabated for ten days or longer.

Treating Allergies

To treat allergies with bee pollen, select a pollen that's pleasing to your palate, because you'll be using a lot of it. During hay fever season or whenever you're exposed to allergens, double, triple, or quadruple your daily bee pollen intake, up to 8 teaspoons maximum per day. Divide your intake and ingest it three to five times per day, each time including 1,000 milligrams of vitamin C (the best and safest natural antihistamine) and a propolis supplement. The idea is to get enough antihistamine and antiallergenic phytochemicals into your body to make a real improvement in acute symptoms.

Some manufacturers sell special bee pollen allergy preparations designed to help acute symptoms. However, they won't help you if you take only one or two capsules per day, because this won't deliver enough of the active phytochemicals and vitamins.

Removing Plantar Warts

Plantar warts are stubborn infections from a papillomavirus that occurs on the base of the foot. When you get one, use the following treatment right away because they can spread. For this remedy you'll need concentrated acetic acid, which is used as an organic weed killer. You can purchase it at home and garden shops and possibly at large natural food stores. You'll only need a little bit of the bottle for the treatment, but the remainder is great to use in the garden because it doesn't harm bees! Alternatively, you can use raw apple cider vinegar or commercial salicylic acid treatment pads, but it may take longer to achieve results. You'll also need propolis capsules, rubbing alcohol, and essential oil of oregano, tea tree, manuka, or cinnamon leaf.

1. After washing your feet with soap (which should be done daily), cut away or file off the top of the wart. Soak a small piece of cotton or gauze in acetic acid and cover the wart. Be forewarned that it will sting! Bandage the area tightly. Repeat this step for 3 days, checking for and cutting off dead tissue each day. Sterilize your cutting tools after each use.

2. On the fourth day, combine the contents of 1 propolis capsule (500 milligrams) with 5 drops of alcohol (either rubbing alcohol or distilled spirits) and 5 drops of oregano oil. (You can substitute tea tree, manuka, or cinnamon leaf oil for the oregano oil.) Mix the ingredients together to make a paste. Apply the paste to the wart and bandage tightly. Repeat for 3 days.

3. Return to step 1 for another 3-day cycle, applying the acetic acid and continuing to cut off dead tissue. Repeat these cycles until the wart no longer has a "cauliflower" appearance and no black spots or roots are visible.

4. If at any point the treated skin becomes very irritated or bleeds a lot, take 3 days off and instead dress the area with raw honey or honey mixed with royal jelly and cover it with a bandage.

TIP: This treatment works for warts on the hands and body, but go very lightly with the acetic acid. These areas are more sensitive than the soles of the feet, where the skin is much thicker and there are fewer nerves close to the surface. It may be advisable to do each step for only 2 days, rather than 3.

Treating Wounds

I often use a combination of raw high desert honey and propolis for wound treatment because it promotes rapid healing and isn't too runny under the bandage. Use a ratio of 1:2 capsules (total about 1 gram) of propolis powder to 1 to 2 tablespoons of raw dark honey.

Raw comb honey with wax and propolis is also an excellent choice because it's thick and tends to stay in place on the wound. Plus, the wax and propolis work with the honey to form a protective antimicrobial seal on the wound.

Simply dip a clean tongue depressor stick or similar applicator or a small utensil into the honey-propolis mixture and spread it over the wound in an even layer. Dress the wound with a large enough bandage that the honey mixture won't squeeze out. Change the bandage twice per day for fresh minor wounds and three times per day for wounds that are large, have become infected, or aren't healing well.

For infected wounds, it's best to soak them in hot salt water for 5 to 10 minutes when you change the dressing; the water should be hot enough that you have to ease into it. You'll be surprised how this helps promote healing. The combination of consistent soaking and dressing the wound with raw honey and propolis will reliably cure infections caused by antibiotic-resistant bacteria.

Another option is to use a propolis salve, which you can purchase at natural food stores, create by mixing propolis into any ointment, or make at home using the formulas on pages 58 and 59. Propolis salves are safe for children and pets. In fact, as pet treatments they have a distinct advantage over ointments based on petroleum jelly: dogs and cats won't enjoy licking a salve with propolis and manuka oil, for example, like they enjoy petroleum jelly.

Propolis-Beeswax WOUND SALVE

This salve is excellent for treating dermatitis, cracked hands, and diaper rash. It incorporates beeswax, which has a long history of use in wound salves, thanks to its healing and anti-inflammatory properties. When melting the beeswax, a candy or meat thermometer can be useful for checking the temperature of the mixture. If using the salve on an infant, don't add tea tree or manuka oil unless you're certain the child isn't allergic to the essential oil.

Heaping ½ teaspoon **propolis powder from capsules**

6 to 8 (10,000 to 25,000 IU) **soft-gel capsules vitamin A**

6 to 8 (400 to 1,000 IU) **soft-gel capsules vitamin D**

4 to 6 (400 IU) **soft-gel capsules vitamin E**

6 (1,000 to 1,300 mg) **soft-gel capsules evening primrose or borage oil**

½ teaspoon **ascorbic acid (vitamin C) powder**

⅛ teaspoon **borax powder**

2 teaspoons **shaved beeswax**

¼ cup **cold-pressed almond, sesame, hazelnut, or olive oil**

2 to 3 teaspoons **glycerin- or ethanol-based liquid herbal extract, such as comfrey, chamomile, yarrow, calendula, or mixed herbs** (optional)

½ teaspoon **tea tree or manuka essential oil** (optional)

Open the propolis capsules into a small dish. Open the capsules of vitamins A, D, and E and evening primrose oil by carefully cutting a slit in each with the tip of a sharp knife. Squeeze the contents into the dish. Add the vitamin C and borax and stir until just combined.

Put the beeswax and almond oil in a small, heavy stainless steel or ceramic saucepan over low heat. Heat, swirling the pan often, until the mixture reaches 175 degrees F (80 degrees C), at which point the melted beeswax will become transparent. Don't let the mixture boil. Remove from the heat and let cool briefly, just until a faint haze of opaque wax forms. Whisk with a small stainless steel whisk until the mixture is fully opaque and has the consistency of very soft butter (100 to 120 degrees F, or 40 to 50 degrees C).

Add the propolis mixture and whisk vigorously and continuously. The mixture will initially soften but then stiffen; when it's still a little soft and warm, but not hot, stir in the herbal extract and optional essential oil. Continue whisking until the mixture is cool. Transfer to small, sterilized containers and seal tightly. Store one container at room temperature, away from heat and light, for immediate use, and refrigerate the others. To use, clean the wound well and dry it thoroughly. Apply a thin layer of the salve, then bandage.

Propolis-Honey BURN AND BLISTER PASTE

When treating wounds, you can simply apply honey first and then sprinkle the propolis from a capsule on top. Alternatively, you can combine these ingredients in a paste for quick application, as in this recipe. This paste is especially effective for burns, abrasions, blisters that have popped, skin ulcers, or inflamed wounds that are healing slowly. Manuka or eucalyptus honey would be especially effective in this recipe, but any dark honey will do. If using this formula to treat burns, including the optional lavender oil will make the paste especially soothing.

1 capsule (1 gram) **propolis powder**

2 tablespoons **raw dark honey**

2 rounded teaspoons **colostrum powder, or** 1 teaspoon **each colostrum powder and freeze-dried royal jelly**

6 drops **manuka, tea tree, eucalyptus, or lavender essential oil** (optional)

Open the propolis capsule into a small dish. Add the honey, colostrum, and optional essential oil and mix to form a smooth but stiff paste. Transfer to a small, sterilized container and seal tightly. Store in a cool, dark place, and avoid getting moisture in the container.

To use the paste, wash the affected area gently and blot dry. Cover with a thin layer of the paste, then wrap with gauze and use first aid tape to hold the dressing in place. Change the dressing twice daily or, if infected, three times daily. At a minimum, clean the wound and apply a fresh dressing each night before you go to bed and let the miracle of propolis and honey work while you sleep!

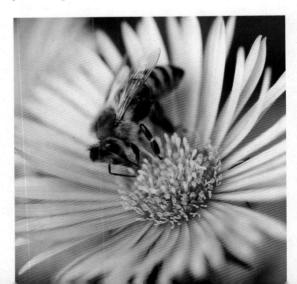

Royal Jelly SKIN TREATMENT GEL

This gel is excellent both for scar treatment and for overall skin protection. When I was pregnant, I used it to prevent stretch marks. It's also great for helping prevent scarring from large wounds or surgery. The recipe calls for sea buckthorn oil, which is red and can stain, so be cautious about getting it or the gel on clothing or other fabrics.

½ cup **100% aloe vera gel**

8 soft-gel (10,000 to 25,000 IU) **capsules vitamin A**

8 soft-gel (400 to 1,000 IU) **capsules vitamin D**

6 (400 IU) **soft-gel capsules vitamin E**

10 (1,000 to 1,300 mg) **soft-gel capsules evening primrose or borage oil**

2 to 3 tablespoons **fresh royal jelly**

2 to 3 teaspoons **sea buckthorn oil**

3 droppers (2 to 3 teaspoons) **calendula extract**

Squeeze or pour the aloe gel into a bottle that holds at least ¾ cup and has a tight-fitting lid. (You need to be able to shake the bottle vigorously.) Open the capsules of vitamins A, D, and E and evening primrose oil by carefully cutting a slit in each with the tip of a sharp knife. Squeeze the contents into the bottle. Add the royal jelly, sea buckthorn oil, and calendula extract and shake thoroughly. If the mixture is too thick to mix effectively, add a few drops of rubbing alcohol or more sea buckthorn oil or calendula extract. Because royal jelly is highly perishable, store the gel in the refrigerator. For short-term use, you can store a small amount in a sterilized jar in a cool, dark place.

To use the gel, first wash the area to be treated. Shake the bottle vigorously, then apply the gel to the area, rubbing it in thoroughly. If using the gel to prevent stretch marks during pregnancy, begin using it at month five. Apply it twice per day, at least once after bathing.

TIPS

- The formula calls for fresh royal jelly. If you only have freeze-dried royal jelly on hand, mix it with a few drops of water and a few drops of rubbing alcohol. Stir well. The royal jelly is rehydrated when it has the consistency of heavy cream. The amount of water and rubbing alcohol needed will depend on the product used and the ambient humidity.

- For an effective sunburn or under-eye treatment (remove contcts before applying), use just the aloe vera gel and royal jelly. Mix well. For drier skin, add the contents of 2 to 4 capsules of evening primrose or borage oil.

- Feel free to experiment with this recipe to create your own personalized skin care treatments.

Propolis THROAT SPRAY AND MOUTH RINSE

Alcohol-based sprays are the best choice for sore throats and preventing respiratory infections, and mouth rinses are the best choice for dental and oral issues. If my throat is scratchy, I like to back up the spray with a few propolis capsules, which contain components that don't dissolve in an extract, no matter what type of solvent is utilized.

20 parts water

1 part ethanol-based propolis extract

Combine the water and propolis extract. Transfer to a glass bottle or spray bottle, and store at room temperature. Use as needed. Increase the ratio of extract to water when a stronger preparation is necessary.

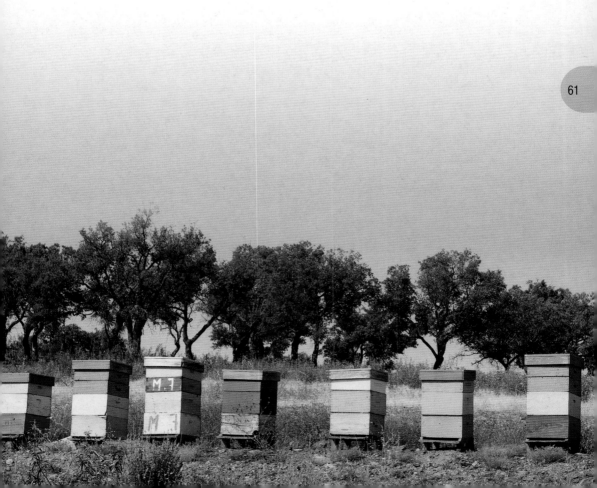

ULCER, GASTRITIS, AND ACID REFLUX *Soother*

If you suffer from an ulcer, gastritis, or acid reflux, you've probably already learned not to go to bed on a full stomach and to avoid alcohol and carbonated beverages late in the evening—or altogether. Taking the following formula at bedtime can also help prevent symptoms and promote healing. If you can find Brazilian green propolis, it will be especially effective in this formula. Alternatively, you can omit the propolis.

2 capsules (1 gram) **propolis powder,** or ½ dropper **propolis extract** (optional)

1 to 2 tablespoons **manuka or buckwheat honey,** preferably raw

2 teaspoons **fresh royal jelly**

Open the propolis capsules into a small dish. Add the honey and royal jelly and mix well. Take the formula on an empty stomach about 20 minutes before retiring, following it with water if you wish. Don't drink anything other than water after taking the formula.

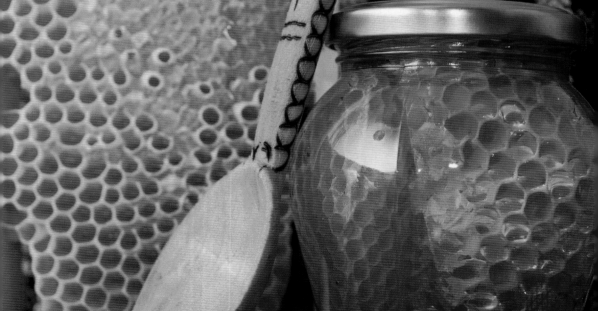

ABOUT THE AUTHOR

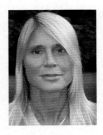

C. Leigh Broadhurst, PhD, is a geochemist and geobotanist for a US government agricultural research center and the Department of Civil and Environmental Engineering, University of Maryland, College Park. She is an expert in environmental remediation and trace elements in the environment and food supply. She has published in the fields of anthropological nutrition, type 2 diabetes, and the role of polyunsaturated fats in human intelligence. Dr. Broadhurst has also been a scientific consultant to the natural products industry for twenty years and is a popular lecturer and talk show guest. She lives in Maryland and North Carolina with her husband, two children, and two dogs.

© 2013 C. Leigh Broadhurst

Photography: Andrew Schmidt, 123RF
Book design, photo editing: John Wincek
Editing: Beth Geisler, Jo Stepaniak

ISBN: 978-1-55312-048-3

Printed in Hong Kong

Published by **Books Alive**
PO Box 99
Summertown, TN 38483
931-964-3571
888-260-8458
www.bookpubco.com

All rights reserved. No portion of this book may be reproduced by any means whatsoever, except for brief quotations in reviews, without written permission from the publisher.

Library of Congress Cataloging-in-Publication Data

Broadhurst, C. Leigh.
  [Health and healing with bee products]
  Bee products for better health / C. Leigh Broadhurst, PhD. — Revised edition.
    pages cm
  Revision of: Health and healing with bee products. — Vancouver, Canada. ; Summertown, Tenn. : Alive Books, 2007.
  Includes bibliographical references.
  ISBN 978-1-55312-048-3 (pbk.) — ISBN 978-1-55312-098-8 (e-book)
 1. Bee products—Therapeutic use. I. Title.
  RM666.B378B76 2013
  638'.16—dc23
                             2012051810

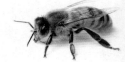

Self-Help Information

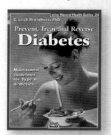 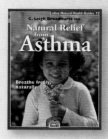 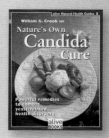

Healthy Recipes

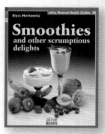 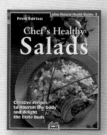 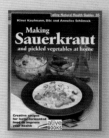

Healing Foods and Herbs

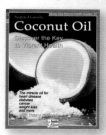 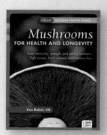 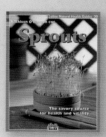

Lifestyles and Alternative Treatments

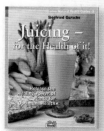 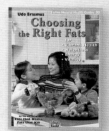 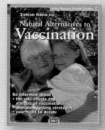

books Alive
Summertown
TENNESSEE

1-800-695-2241 • www.healthy-eating.com